LEAN IN
15

THE SUSTAIN PLAN

JOE
WICKS

The Body Coach

First published 2016 by Bluebird
an imprint of Pan Macmillan
20 New Wharf Road, London N1 9RR
Associated companies throughout the world
www.panmacmillan.com

ISBN 978-1-5098-2022-1

Grateful acknowledgement is made to 'My Lean Winners' and the 'Lean in 15 Heroes'
for permission to include the images on pages 224–33 and 238–9.

Credits
Publisher: Carole Tonkinson
Design: Ami Smithson
Desk Editor: Claire Gatzen
Food Photography: Maja Smend
Fitness Photography: Glen Burrows
Food Styling: Bianca Nice
Prop Styling: Lydia Brun

9 8 7 6 5 4

A CIP catalogue record for this book is available from the British Library.

Printed in Italy

Designed and Typeset by www.cabinlondon.co.uk

Visit www.panmacmillan.com to read more about all our books and to buy them.
You will also find features, author interviews and news of any author events, and you
can sign up for e-newsletters so that you're always first to hear about our new releases.

Bluebird publish books bringing you the very latest in diet,
self-help and popular psychology, as well as parenting, career
and business, and memoir.

We make books for life in every sense: life-enhancing but also
lasting; the ones you will turn to again and again for inspiration.

For 10 extra Lean in 15 recipes and to hear more about
Bluebird visit www.TheBodyCoachBooks.com

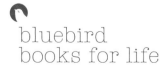

CONTENTS

//

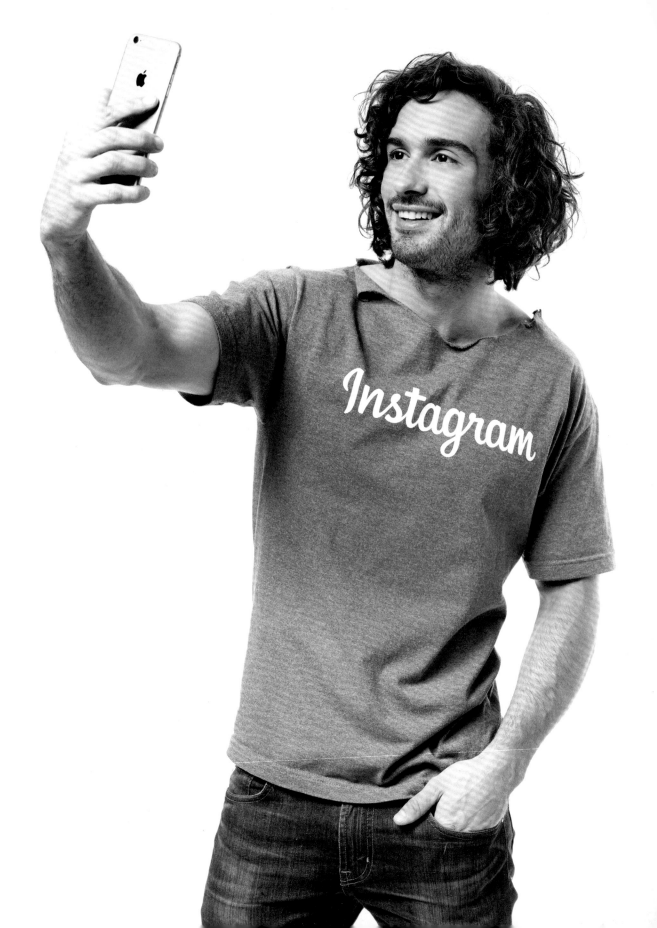

INTRODUCTION

//

Wow, what an incredible year it's been for Lean in 15! I still can't quite believe that something that started out as a bit of fun on social media has gone on to inspire and help so many people. It's been a real rollercoaster twelve months for me, from singing to midget trees out of my kitchen window in Surbiton to having a bestselling cookbook translated into more than seventeen languages.

> **' I owe my success to my social media followers '**

I want to start with a thank you because I know I owe my success to my social media followers. You are the ones who have given me your time and attention and have been with me on my journey. Without you, I wouldn't have been given a book deal and, because of your willingness to like, comment on and share my recipes, you made my books record breakers. Thanks for all your support and for helping me get my message out to the world.

My goal when I began sharing recipes online was simple: to get people cooking healthy food and to make it as easy as possible, which in my opinion is the key to fat-loss success. The less hassle you have in the kitchen, the more likely you are to stick to a plan.

As a nation, we are now working longer hours than ever and it has led many of us to believe that we simply don't have enough time to stop and cook healthy meals. In reality, this is just an excuse we've all used at some point or other to skip meals and grab fast food on the go – and it's a big barrier that I want to help you break through.

With Lean in 15 you'll see just how easy it is to cook your own healthy meals and start not only to regain control of your body but also to form the habits that will help you sustain a lean body all year round.

Instagram is where the idea for Lean in 15 began, but I never imagined I would end up cooking live on TV or writing a book. Can you imagine how excited I was when one day I got an email from my (now) publisher asking if I wanted to come in for a meeting? To be honest, I thought it was a joke at first, but it turns out they were serious – and here I am, sitting in my flat, writing my third book in just over a year.

I remember the day I signed the book deal so clearly. I called my mum straight afterwards and screamed down the phone, 'Mum, you won't believe it – I'm going to write a book!' I ended up laughing and crying because I was so overwhelmed and happy. You never forget those moments. Just like the time I was walking down the street and she said, 'Joe, one day I'm going to see your face on the side of a bus.' I laughed and replied, 'Don't be silly, Mum, why would anyone want to see my face on a bus?' A few months later, just as she'd predicted, there it was – my face on a Lean in 15 poster driving past us down Oxford Street. I guess it's true what they say: mums are always right!

I still to this day laugh when my mates see me on TV and ask, 'Joe, how on earth have you become a TV chef?' My answer is always the same: 'Sssh, don't tell anyone I'm not a chef.' The truth is, I'm just a personal trainer who loves to cook. I'm completely self-taught in the kitchen so there are no Michelin stars hanging on my wall. This has proved to be a good thing, though, because it means my meals are really quick and easy to make, and even if you're a complete beginner you'll be able to follow my recipes. The vast majority of the meals can be made in 15 minutes, so they're perfect for busy people who don't have hours to spend in the kitchen every day. There are a few that take a bit longer, but they taste amazing and are worth the wait. All the ingredients can be found in your local supermarket and many meals can be batch-cooked for the week ahead, so fitting Lean in 15 into your lifestyle is a doddle.

I believe good nutrition doesn't need to be complicated and staying lean doesn't need to be difficult. I'm all about keeping it simple and taking it back to basics, with straightforward, nutrient-dense foods to fuel your body. After all, results come with consistency, so if you love the food you eat each day and don't go hungry, you'll find it much easier to achieve the body you want.

I'm really excited to share this third instalment of Lean in 15 with you. Book 1, *The Shift Plan*, and Book 2, *The Shape Plan*, have already helped thousands of people get fitter, leaner and healthier, and I'm confident this book will do the same for you.

I find it utterly amazing to see so many people following my recipes and workouts. Nothing makes me happier than to hear stories from people who have used my advice to get healthier, and it only makes me more motivated to keep doing what I do. I truly am a man on a mission to get the world lean and off fad diets once and for all.

The aim of the Sustain Plan is to get you fitter, stronger and leaner but, more importantly, to show you how to maintain your results long into the future. I want you to know that this isn't one of those low-calorie recipe books promising quick results. I don't believe in them because they don't work over the long term. My goal with this book is to show you how to fuel your body with the right foods at the right time, so that you stay lean all year round. I don't want you to spend another day on restricted calories or another year yo-yo dieting. This book is going to help you change your approach to nutrition, and show you that you can eat much more food than you think and still stay lean.

I'm also going to introduce you to a new training method which I call Pyramid Resistance HIIT. This is where you will combine a form of weight training with high intensity interval training to get your body building lean muscle and burning fat for fun.

Thank you for buying my third book and good luck on your journey to becoming a lean winner. If you commit to the Lean in 15 lifestyle and stay consistent with your training and nutrition, you will achieve the body you want this year. Go get it.

Keep it Lean.

Joe Wicks

> 'THE AIM OF THE SUSTAIN PLAN IS TO GET YOU STRONGER AND LEANER AND TO MAINTAIN YOUR RESULTS'

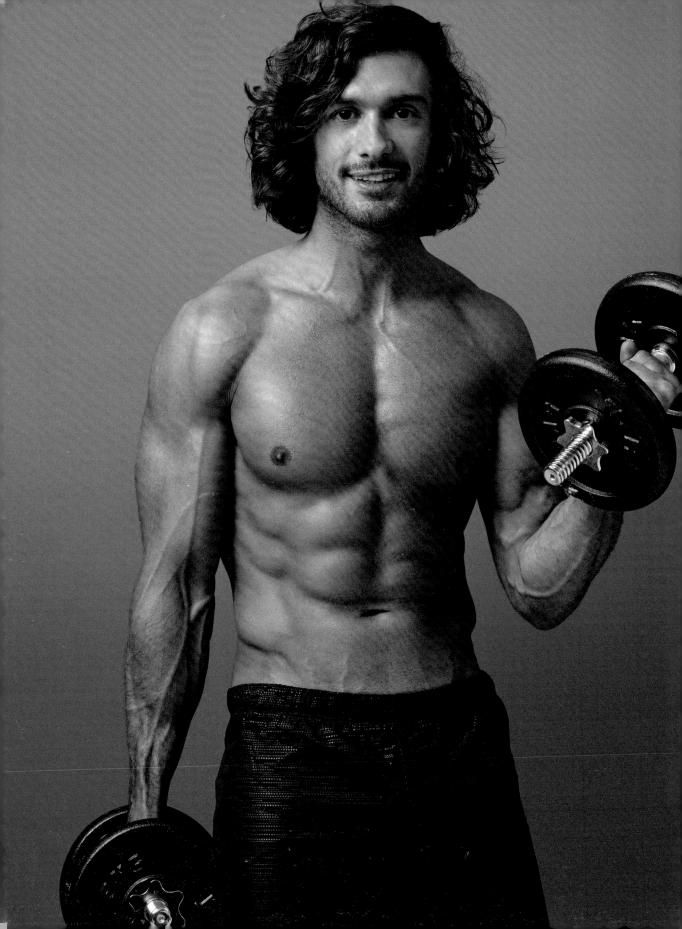

THE
LEAN IN 15
SUSTAIN
PLAN

FUELLING YOUR BODY FOR SUCCESS

//

Welcome to *Lean in 15 – The Sustain Plan*. This is the final phase taken from my 90 Day Shift, Shape and Sustain Plan, my tailored online programme which is transforming thousands of people around the world every day.

Although the training and meal structure in this book is similar to my online plan, it's important for me to point out that these recipes are not individually tailored to your body. This would be impossible, as everyone has a different body type and energy demands.

You may find, therefore, that the portions in this book are perfect, too large or too small for you, depending on your appetite and your daily activity levels. The only way you can really find this out is by giving it a go and seeing how you feel. I always say to my clients: you should eat to feel awesome. If you are physically active in your job and train hard five days per week then clearly you will require more energy than someone who is more sedentary. The key here is to listen to your body and not to go hungry. If you feel the food portions are not providing you with enough energy, simply increase them, and vice versa if you feel too full.

You'll notice that I don't display the calories in my recipes. This is because I want you to break away from numbers-based thinking; I don't believe people should go hungry or obsess over daily calorie targets. That's not enjoyable and it's not fun. I want you to keep it simple, and to focus more on the type and quality of the foods you're eating and on when you're eating in relation to your exercise. Once you combine my nutritious recipes with regular exercise, you'll soon start to see positive changes in your body.

Please don't be drawn into the old way of thinking that you need to drastically cut calories to make your body burn fat. We know this doesn't work in the long run because the body needs energy to burn fat. In fact, the body's greatest energy demand – around 70 per cent – comes from its resting metabolic rate, so massively undereating and depriving your body of calories means it stands no chance of getting lean.

You need to create only a very small energy deficit to kick-start your metabolism into burning fat. I've purposefully created quite high-calorie meals because the training is very intense and you're going to need lots of energy. If, however, you do feel the portion sizes are too much and you're not making progress, just reduce them slightly until you start to see progress.

Ultimately, the aim of this plan is to get you eating more food so you can ditch low-calorie diets for good. When you learn to fuel your body correctly you can get lean and sustain your results. There's no quick fix, though. It's going to take time, dedication and consistency to build the body you want.

What makes the Sustain Plan different?

The meal structure in this plan returns to that of my first book, *The Shift Plan*, where you will be following my post-workout carbohydrate-refuel method. This way of eating is very effective for fat loss, as it will ensure your body is utilizing the right energy source at the right time and in line with its energy demands. Put simply, you will be eating more carbohydrates around your workouts on training days and then reducing them on rest days in exchange for healthy fats. The training plan is completely new.

Remember, though, that there is NO single perfect eating plan for everyone. Here's a quick outline of the different plans:

'I WANT YOU TO BREAK AWAY FROM NUMBERS-BASED THINKING'

THE SHIFT PLAN
EATING STRUCTURE

On a training day you will consume two reduced-carbohydrate meals and one post-workout carbohydrate-refuel meal, as well as two snacks.

On a rest day you will consume three reduced-carbohydrate meals and two snacks.

THE SHAPE PLAN
EATING STRUCTURE

On a training day in this phase you will consume three carbohydrate-rich meals and two snacks.

On a rest day you will consume three reduced-carbohydrate meals and two snacks.

As you can see, in Book 2, *The Shape Plan*, I encouraged you to eat three carbohydrate-rich meals on a training day. This was because I wanted you to establish for yourself whether your body runs better on a higher-carb diet or a higher-fat diet. Personally, I feel awesome and full of energy eating two reduced-carbohydrate meals per day and one big post-workout carbohydrate-refuel meal, as described in this book.

If, however, you have more energy, train harder and recover quicker when eating three carbohydrate-rich meals per day, then that is exactly what you should do. My advice is to eat to feel energized, so give the Sustain Plan eating structure a go for a month and see how you feel. If you feel lethargic then simply increase your carb intake and try having two refuel meals and one reduced-carbohydrate meal per day.

How will I be eating on the Sustain Plan?

The recipes in this book are broken down into three sections: reduced-carbohydrate meals, post-workout carbohydrate-refuel meals, and snacks and treats.

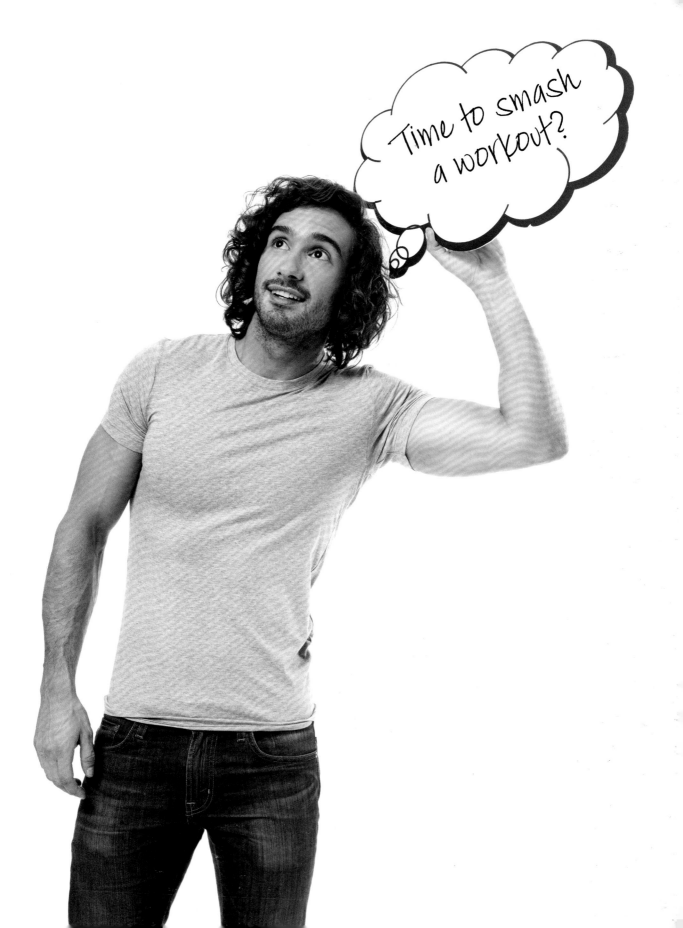

On a training day you will consume two reduced-carbohydrate meals and one post-workout carbohydrate-refuel meal as well as two snacks.

On a rest day you will consume three reduced-carbohydrate meals and two snacks.

All the meals are interchangeable, which means that on a training day you can eat any of the post-workout refuel meals at any time of the day. For example, you can have the protein pancakes (page 109) after you train in the morning for breakfast, or, alternatively, for dinner if you train in the evening.

Regardless of how late you train in the evening, always remember to have your post-workout refuel meal afterwards. This is important because during intense exercise you will deplete your muscles of their stored carbohydrates (glycogen), and so you'll need to top them up. This ensures your muscles can be repaired and refuelled ready for your next workout.

How is the training different?

The training plan in this book is a progression from Books 1 and 2. You will be introduced to Pyramid Resistance HIIT, which is even more intense than the Volume Resistance HIIT in *The Shape Plan*. If you are a complete beginner, I recommend building up your fitness first with some of my free YouTube workouts (The Body Coach TV) before attempting the training in this book.

> **Lack of sleep could be the one thing holding you back**

How can a good night's sleep help me get lean?

Many people underestimate the importance of sleep when it comes to burning fat and building lean muscle. There are a few reasons why a lack of sleep can slow down or halt your fat loss – some are more obvious than others. This could be the one thing holding you back from making progress.

There is a strong link between the amount of sleep you get and your performance when you exercise. After a poor night's sleep, you'll instantly notice that the intensity of your workouts will drop dramatically. You may not even have the motivation or energy to train, so you might find yourself hitting the snooze button and skipping your workouts altogether. If this happens every day, you could end up going weeks without completing a decent workout. Turning the TV off and getting your head on the pillow an hour earlier than you're used to really will make a huge difference to your body over time.

Another common side effect of a sleep-deprived night, which I'm sure you will have experienced, is a craving for sugary foods. I personally want to eat every single carb I can get my hands on after a rough night's sleep – bagels, crumpets, muffins, toast . . . Not only will your body crave sugar, but your appetite will also increase and you'll want to consume way more food than normal. When you combine a lack of exercise with an increase in calorie intake from junk food, it's easy to see why sleep can have a huge impact on your body fat levels.

Here are my top tips for a deep sleep. These have really helped me to improve the quality of my sleep, be more productive, train harder and get leaner.

- **Stay off social media.** Switch off your laptop and mobile at least 30 minutes before bed and leave them in another room. Let your bedroom be a sanctuary.

- **Ditch the bedroom TV.** Get yourself a DAB radio alarm clock instead. Playing some mellow tunes always helps me to fall asleep and makes me feel so happy when I wake up.

- **Go dark.** Get yourself a comfortable eye mask. It takes getting used to at first but trust me, this really will allow you to sleep deeper and longer because the early morning sun won't wake you up.

- **Get into a routine.** Aim to fall asleep at the same time each day so that your body's internal clock runs smoothly.

Mind over mattress

When you've mastered your sleep, you can harness your energy and win the battle of the bed every morning. You'll wake up and be ready to nail your workouts, prep like a boss and win the day.

FORMING NEW HABITS

2

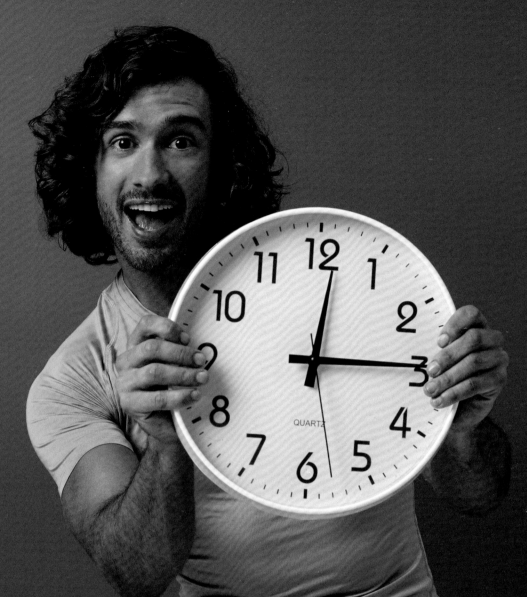

FORMING
NEW
HABITS

The hardest part of sticking to a fitness and nutrition plan is committing for the long haul, but once you get going, new habits will form and create a momentum that will carry you forward.

In case this is the first book of mine you've picked up, I'll quickly review the basics.

The first thing you're going to need to do in order to make this plan work for you is pick up a few essential items:

- **A mountain of food storage containers – to store all your prepped meals**

- **A set of digital food scales – to weigh your ingredients out and maintain portion control**

- **A decent wok or pan – because there's nothing worse than a sticky one**

- **A small food processor or blender – to make smoothies, sauces and pesto**

- **A bench and set of dumbbells** – only if you plan on training at home

- **A refillable water bottle** – to ensure you consume enough water each day

I'll start it tomorrow

Once you have the essential items, you'll have all the kit you need to complete this plan and become a lean winner.

You might now hear that voice in your head that says, 'I'll start it tomorrow.' We've all listened to it before and it's often the thing that delays or prevents us from achieving our health and fitness goals.

But let's not listen to it today – let's get motivated and set the ball rolling. It may seem daunting embarking on a new nutrition and exercise regime, but once you begin to feel the benefits and see the results, you'll wish you'd started sooner.

How do you stay motivated?

On social media and when I give talks, people often ask: 'Joe, how do you stay motivated to eat well and exercise?' The truth is, I've always loved exercise, even as a kid, so for me that part is easy. Working out makes me feel good. It gives me energy, keeps me focused and boosts my confidence. This is how I always want to feel, so for me personally it's a case of, why would I not do it?

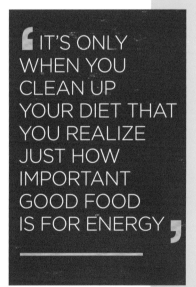

IT'S ONLY WHEN YOU CLEAN UP YOUR DIET THAT YOU REALIZE JUST HOW IMPORTANT GOOD FOOD IS FOR ENERGY

Nutrition, on the other hand, has not always been easy for me. Like most people, I was addicted to sugar. I loved cereal, fizzy drinks and chocolate bars and was pretty lazy when it came to cooking. But the day I started to really study nutrition and cut the junk out of my life, I instantly understood why it was so important.

So many people plod along with their poor diet and eating habits, convinced that it's normal to feel tired and lethargic all the time. It's only when you clean up your diet and remove fast food, processed meals and refined sugars that you realize just how important good food is for energy and wellbeing.

I choose to eat the way I do now because I want to have energy. Real energy from real food, so that I can wake up, smash a workout, work really hard and feel full of energy all day. Once you get that feeling of being energized and productive all day long, it's easy to want it all the time, and the temptation to eat junk food really does start to disappear.

Remember, keep taking progress pics and don't be tempted to get back on the sad step (my name for bathroom scales). Numbers do not tell the whole truth – progress pics and how you feel are much better indicators.

It won't happen overnight, though: it may take you weeks or even months to properly shake off your cravings, but when you do you'll feel awesome.

Help, I've had a blowout!

If I do have a blowout and binge on a takeaway, loads of fizzy drinks and chocolate or sweets, or even knock back a few drinks, I'm literally knackered for the whole day and normally the next day too. My digestive system takes a beating; I'm tired and low on energy. It's because of this feeling that I choose to live the Lean in 15 lifestyle.

If you do wake up feeling jaded on the back of a day of bad eating, I would recommend making yourself get up and smash a workout. You won't feel like it, but it's the best way to ensure that a day of bad eating doesn't become a week of bad eating.

Don't forget to stay hydrated: it's key to getting you back on track. I aim for between 2 and 4 litres of water per day.

Don't forget to stay hydrated: it's key to getting you back on track

What to do if you're travelling

This is something else I get asked a lot by people who travel frequently or have very social jobs. Check out my YouTube channel, The Body Coach TV, for hotel workouts. You can smash out a full workout even in the smallest of hotel rooms – no gym necessary.

When you're eating in a restaurant, try to make smart choices and keep it simple. Steer clear of the breakfast bar, which will try to tempt you with pastries and sugary drinks. Instead, stick to eggs, simply prepared (poached, boiled or scrambled), toast if you've worked out, and a nice black coffee. During the day, lean meats or fish with a simple side salad or steamed greens are perfect. For me, nothing beats a grilled steak and leafy green salad – something most restaurants will be able to provide.

If you're going to be lured by the minibar, take some healthy snacks with you – raw, unsweetened nuts such as almonds are great energy boosters and will make sure you don't get stuck into the Pringles.

Winners o'clock

You may have heard the social media saying, 'Set your alarm for winners o'clock.' I've been asked many times when that time actually is! LOL. It isn't actually a specific time. Winners o'clock could be 6am, 9pm, or any time for that matter. Winners o'clock is when you set aside some time to do your workout and achieve success. It's when you walk away a winner.

There is no optimal time to work out so I always advise my clients to train when they have the most energy and also when it suits their lifestyle.

	MONDAY	TUESDAY	WEDNESDAY	THURSDAY	FRIDAY	SATURDAY	SUNDAY
Training am	Chest and back		Rest day	Legs	Rest day		Rest day
Post-workout	Joe's protein shake			Joe's protein shake			
Meal 1	Quinoa overnight oats	Smoky omelette	'Nutella' smoothie	Spiced turkey and beans on toast	Vanilla and mango tahini smoothie	No-bread Benedict	Salmon and avocado sesame egg roll
Snack	Boiled egg	Apple	75g blueberries	30g nuts	Boiled egg	Apple	Roasted cauliflower hummus
Meal 2	Cheat's chicken Caesar	Cauliflower rice with coconut prawns	Chicken caprese	Bacon, leek and pea frittata	Sammy sea bass with crunchy carrots	Sea bass with lemon and fennel coleslaw	Joe's beef and mushroom pie
Snack	30g nuts	Quinoa and carrot fritters	Cheat's taramasalata	75g blueberries	Cheat's taramasalata	85g beef jerky	30g nuts
Training pm		Arms				Shoulders and abs	
Post-workout		Joe's protein shake				Joe's protein shake	
Meal 3	Cajun salmon	Thai beef noodle salad	Moroccan monkfish	Duck rendang	Massaman curry	Sausage and mushroom penne pasta	Chicken salad with lemon pesto

My Shape Plan perfect week

• • • • • • • • • • • • • • • •

I've created this table to show you a typical week for me, using the recipes and the workouts in this book. Hopefully it will give you some ideas to plan your own week. Use the table opposite to help you prep like a boss.

	MONDAY	TUESDAY	WEDNESDAY	THURSDAY	FRIDAY	SATURDAY	SUNDAY
Training am							
Post-workout							
Meal 1							
Snack							
Meal 2							
Snack							
Training pm							
Post-workout							
Meal 3							

USE THIS TABLE TO PLAN YOUR OWN MEALS AND WORKOUTS FOR THE WEEK

Prepping like a boss
. . . .

The quickest route to successful fat loss in my and my clients' experience is being able to take control of your diet, and this means cooking and preparing your own meals as much as possible. By prepping your meals at the weekend or the night before work you are setting yourself up for success, because you know exactly what you will be eating and can avoid junk food on the go. You'll not only burn fat quicker and get results faster; you'll also save money in the long run because you won't be spending so much eating out every day.

REDUCED-CARBOHYDRATE RECIPES

3

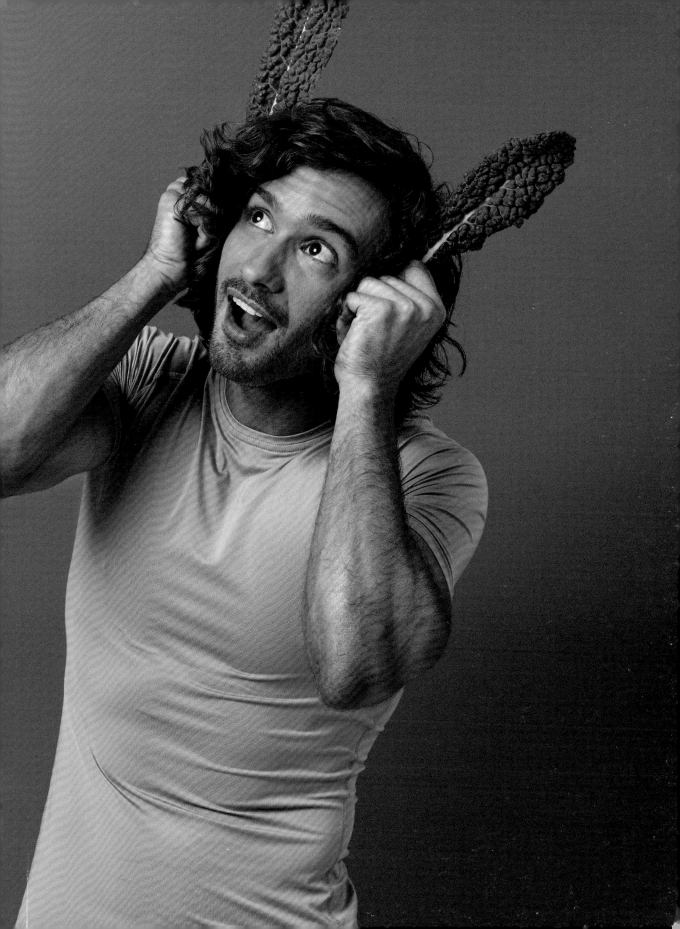

50g blanched hazelnuts
300ml almond milk
1 tbsp drinking chocolate
2 scoops (60g) chocolate
  protein powder
1 tbsp hazelnut butter

★ Chocolate protein powders
have different strengths:
go for a lighter, milk
chocolate to avoid bitterness.

100g blueberries
100ml coconut milk
100ml almond milk
small handful of ice
50g reduced-fat Greek yoghurt
2 scoops (60g) vanilla protein
  powder

75g mango chunks
175ml almond milk
small handful of ice
2 scoops (60g) vanilla protein
  powder
25g tahini
tiny sprinkle of salt
squeeze of fresh lime juice

'NUTELLA' SMOOTHIE

Everybody loves Nutella, right? Well, so far I've never met anyone who doesn't. This smoothie tastes like the naughty treat, but fills you full of good fats. Make sure you toast the hazelnuts to really bring out the flavour.

METHOD

Toast the hazelnuts in a dry pan until they are golden brown all over. Tip them onto a chopping board and roughly chop into small pieces.

Scrape the hazelnuts into a blender and pour in just a splash of the milk and all the remaining ingredients. Blitz until smooth.

Add the remaining milk to the blender and blitz one last time to bring everything together.

Pour out the smoothie and get it down you.

BLUEBERRY AND COCONUT SMOOTHIE

Another super-tasty smoothie that's great to grab once a week, especially if you're in a mad rush. Try not to rely on smoothies every day, though. Focus on eating three large meals instead to ensure your body is fuelled properly.

METHOD

Chuck all the ingredients into a blender and blitz until smooth.

VANILLA AND MANGO TAHINI SMOOTHIE

This smoothie is perfect if you want something quick on the go. Make sure you eat a wide selection of recipes from the book to ensure you get all the nutrients your body needs.

METHOD

Place all the ingredients in a blender and blitz until smooth.

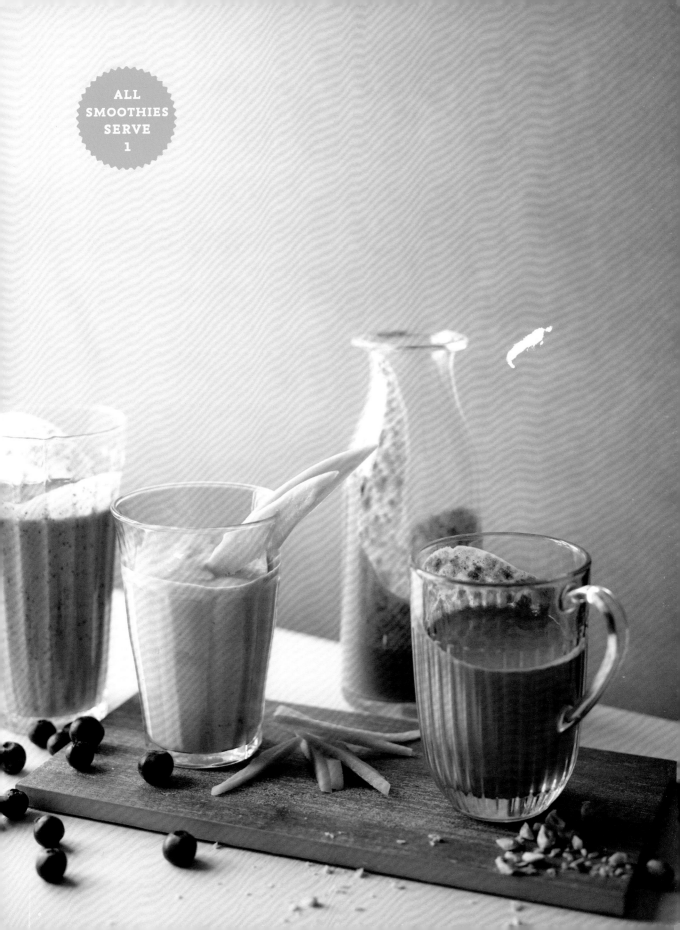

BACON, LEEK AND PEA FRITTATA

SERVES 2

REDUCED-CARB
MAKE AHEAD

INGREDIENTS

1 tsp butter
½ leek, trimmed, washed and
    finely shredded
4 rashers of back bacon,
    sliced into 1cm strips
45g frozen peas
6 eggs
salt and pepper
1 ball of mozzarella (roughly
    125g drained), torn into large
    chunks
1 ripe avocado, sliced
small green salad, to serve
25g pine nuts, to serve –
    optional

Ooooh! I do love a frittata. They're so easy to make and can be eaten hot or cold. This one has bacon so you know it's going to taste good. You can even prep the night before and have it ready to reheat in a few minutes.

METHOD

Preheat your grill to maximum.

Melt the butter in a medium non-stick frying pan over a medium to high heat. When bubbling, add the leek and bacon and fry for about 3 minutes, or until the bacon is cooked through and the leek softened.

Add the frozen peas and cook for about 1 minute, or until they have defrosted.

Beat the eggs together with a little salt and black pepper. Crank up the heat to maximum under the pan and, when the butter is bubbling up, pour in the eggs and cook, pulling the edges into the middle as they start to set.

When most of the egg is cooked, scatter over the mozzarella and slide your pan under the hot grill – if you have a pan with a plastic handle then make sure it doesn't end up under the element. Cook for about 3 minutes, or until the egg is totally set and the mozzarella melted and bubbling.

Slide the frittata from the pan and cut into wedges. Serve with the avocado slices, a small side salad and a scattering of pine nuts, if you like.

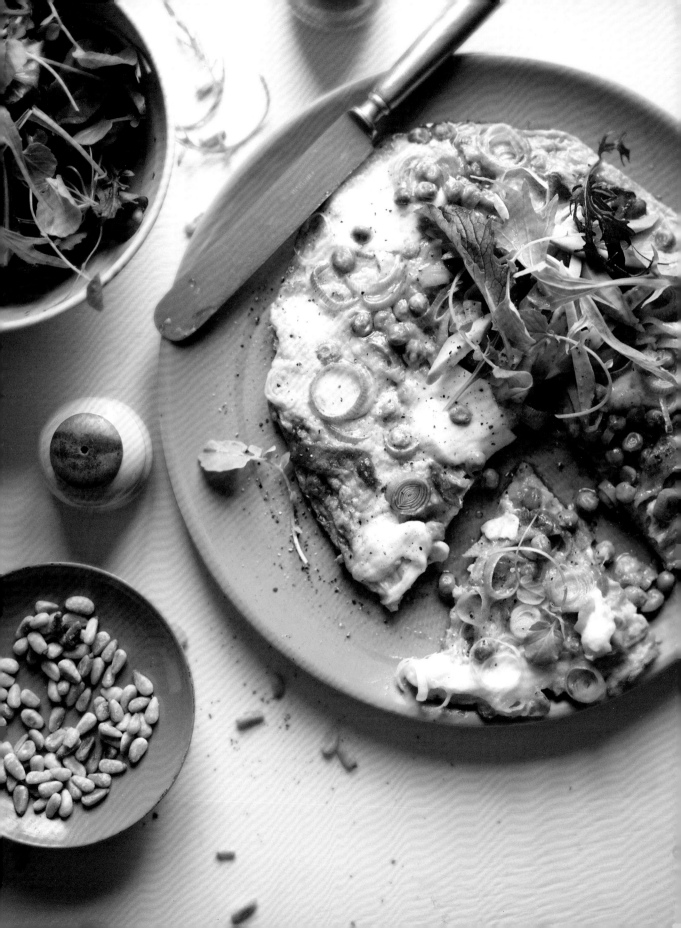

RED PEPPER MUSHROOMS WITH AVOCADO

SERVES 1

INGREDIENTS

½ tbsp coconut oil
2 spring onions, finely sliced
6 chestnut mushrooms,
   roughly quartered
1 jarred red pepper, drained
   and sliced into 1cm strips
40g tinned chickpeas, drained
   and rinsed
1 ripe avocado, de-stoned
juice of 1 lime
1 red chilli, de-seeded and
   finely sliced
salt and pepper
25g feta
15g pumpkin seeds

Here's a nice little vegetarian breakfast for you to try. It's not rammed with protein but it's got plenty of healthy fats, so it'll provide you with lots of energy for the day ahead.

METHOD

Melt the coconut oil in a large frying pan over a medium to high heat. Add the spring onions and chestnut mushrooms and fry, stirring only occasionally, for about 2 minutes.

Chuck in the red pepper and chickpeas along with about 1 tablespoon of water, and stir-fry for 2 minutes, by which time the mushrooms and chickpeas should be cooked through. Turn off the heat from under the pan.

Scoop the avocado flesh into a bowl and add the lime juice and red chilli along with a good pinch of salt and pepper. Use the back of a fork to smash everything together until well combined.

Spoon the mushroom mix onto a plate, dollop on the avocado, crumble over the feta and finish with a scattering of crunchy pumpkin seeds.

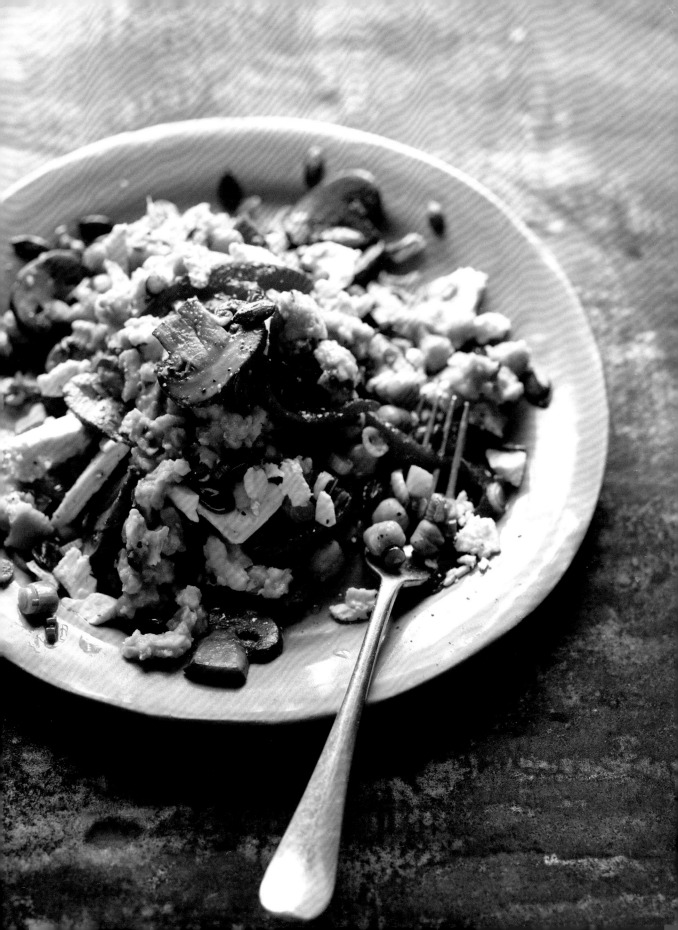

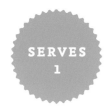

SMOKY OMELETTE

This is proper tasty breakfast fuel. Ditch the sugary cereals if you want to get lean this year and give this a go instead. RIP body fat!

REDUCED-CARB INGREDIENTS

1 tsp butter
1 rasher of streaky smoked bacon, sliced into 1cm strips
100g skinless smoked haddock, chopped into 1cm chunks
3 spring onions, finely sliced
3 eggs
25ml double cream
salt and pepper
large handful of baby spinach leaves
20g cheddar, grated
large handful of rocket or watercress, to serve

METHOD

Melt the butter in a medium frying pan over a medium to high heat. When bubbling, add the bacon, smoked haddock and spring onions. Fry, stirring regularly, for 1 minute.

Meanwhile, whisk up the eggs with the double cream and a good pinch of salt and pepper.

Load the baby spinach into the frying pan with the bacon and fish and stir it about until it has completely wilted.

Crank up the heat to maximum and pour in the beaten eggs. Make your omelette by carefully drawing in the cooked edges to the centre. Repeat until pretty much all of the egg is cooked and there is only a little loose egg on top.

Sprinkle over the cheddar and then fold the omelette in half, making a half-moon shape.

Slide the omelette onto a plate, top with a small mountain of salad leaves and get stuck in.

SALMON AND AVOCADO SESAME EGG ROLL

SERVES 1

REDUCED-CARB
MAKE AHEAD

INGREDIENTS

2 eggs
3 tsp sesame seed oil
2 tsp coconut oil
1 ripe avocado, de-stoned
1 red chilli, de-seeded and finely sliced
¼ cucumber, diced
2 spring onions, finely sliced
2 tsp rice wine vinegar
125g smoked salmon, roughly chopped
salt and pepper
small handful of watercress
15g pumpkin seeds

This is not an omelette! Well, it sort of is, but actually what you're after is a much thinner egg base than an omelette. Sesame oil may seem weird in this recipe, but trust me, it goes perfectly with the avocado and salmon.

METHOD

Crack the eggs into a bowl and beat together with half of the sesame seed oil.

Melt the coconut oil in a large frying pan over a high heat. Pour in the egg mixture, spreading it as thinly and evenly as possible over the base of the pan. Fry for about 30 seconds, then flip and give it another 30 seconds. Slide the thin egg base from the frying pan and leave to one side until ready to use.

Scoop the avocado flesh into a bowl and add the chilli, cucumber, spring onions, vinegar, smoked salmon and the rest of the sesame seed oil, along with a good pinch of salt and pepper. Use the back of a fork or a wooden spoon to smash everything together until well mixed.

Lay the thin 'omelette' on a plate, spoon on the salmon mix, top with watercress, scatter with the pumpkin seeds and then roll up tightly. This is now perfect to wrap up in some tin foil and take to work for your lunch.

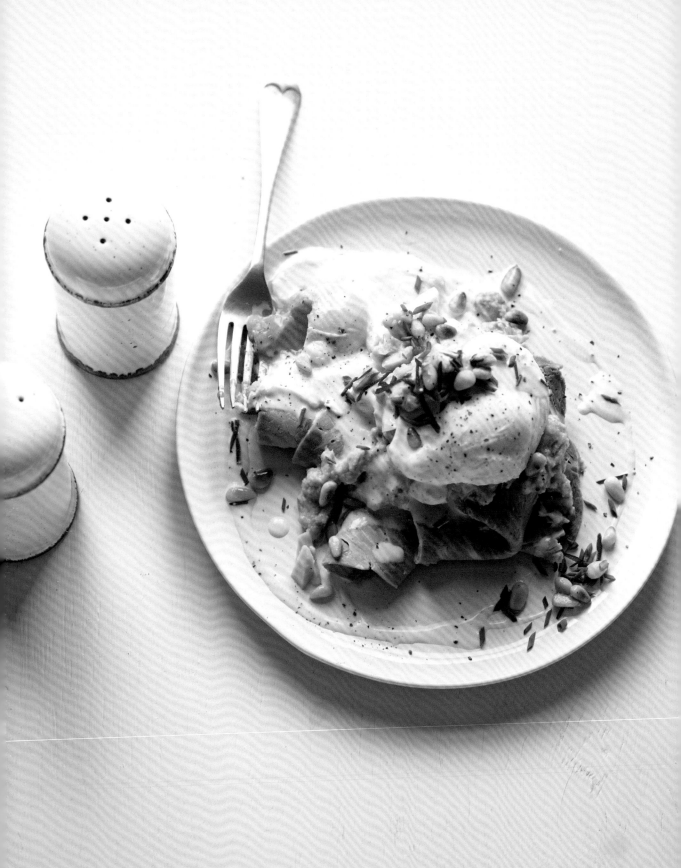

NO-BREAD BENEDICT

SERVES 1

REDUCED-CARB INGREDIENTS

1 ripe avocado, de-stoned
salt and pepper
2 thick slices of deli-style ham
  (about 130g)
2 eggs
2 tbsp mayonnaise
1 tsp Dijon mustard
2 tsp white wine vinegar
10g pine nuts
sprinkling of chopped chives –
  optional
1 red chilli, de-seeded and
  finely sliced – optional

Well that's brunch sorted, then. There may not be a big muffin underneath but this still tastes banging. Make sure you get some decent thick-sliced, deli-style ham and not the cheap wafer-thin stuff.

METHOD

Bring a saucepan of water to the boil.

Meanwhile, scoop the avocado flesh into a bowl, season with salt and pepper and smash up with the back of a fork. Leave to one side.

Lay the ham slices on a microwaveable plate, sprinkle with water, cover with cling film and zap in the microwave for about 1 minute or until hot. Leave under the cling film until you're ready to eat.

Your water should be boiling by now, so carefully crack in the eggs and poach at a gentle simmer for about 4 minutes for a runny yolk.

While the eggs are poaching, make your hollandaise sauce: whisk together the mayonnaise, mustard and vinegar along with 3 tablespoons of warm water (I just spoon a bit of the poaching water straight in).

Now start building your brekkie. Lay the ham on a plate, pile on the smashed avocado, top with the poached eggs and spoon over the hollandaise. Finish with a sprinkling of pine nuts, and chives and red chilli, if using.

This is good – really good.

REDUCED-CARB
GOOD TO FREEZE
INGREDIENTS

½ tbsp coconut oil
2 star anise
240g skinless duck breast
  fillet, sliced into 1cm strips
2 cloves garlic, finely chopped
1 lemongrass stalk, tender
  white part only, finely sliced
2 tbsp red curry paste
125ml coconut milk
2 tbsp desiccated coconut
handful of coriander, roughly
  chopped
lime wedges, to serve

★ Serve with a pile of
midget trees (tender-stem
broccoli) and spinach or
green beans.

DUCK RENDANG

Curries are one of my favourite things in the world so I had to include a new one in this book. I use red curry paste because it's easy to find in supermarkets and tastes amazing with duck.

METHOD

Melt the coconut oil in a large frying pan or wok over a high heat. Add the star anise and fry for 30 seconds on its own.

Next chuck in the duck, garlic and lemongrass and stir-fry for 1 minute, which should be enough time for the duck to brown. Dollop in the curry paste and toss to coat all the ingredients.

Reduce the heat to medium and slowly pour in the coconut milk, stirring to work the paste into the milk until it becomes a sauce. Crank up the heat one last time and simmer the curry for 2 minutes, or until you are happy the duck is cooked through (although it is perfectly safe to cat duck rare).

Remove the pan from the heat, stir in the desiccated coconut and coriander and serve up with lime wedges to squeeze over.

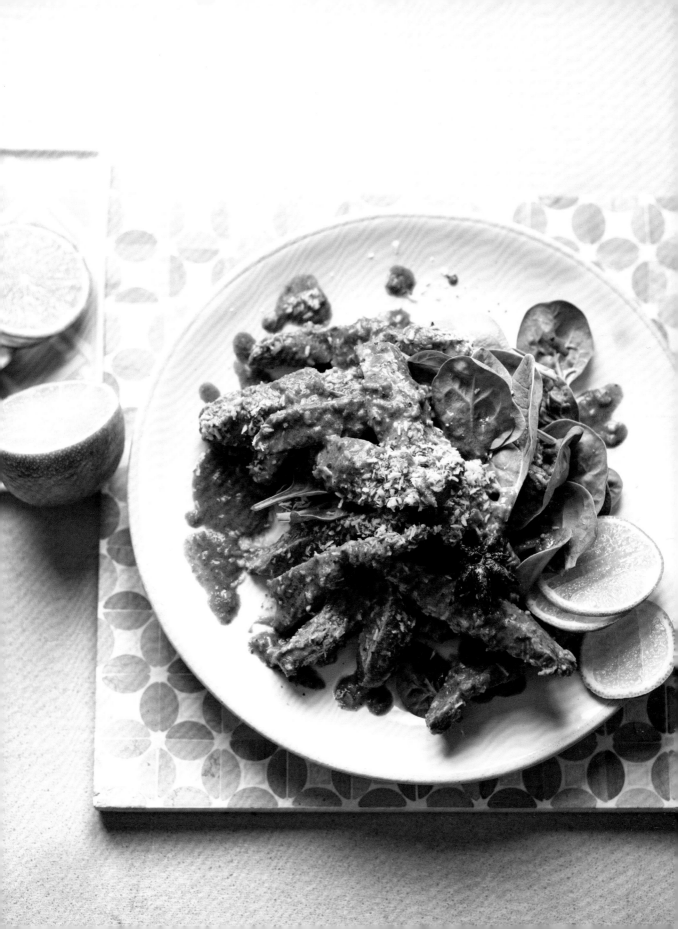

TURMERIC CHICKEN WITH SPINACH SATAY

SERVES 1

REDUCED-CARB
MAKE AHEAD
INGREDIENTS

1 x 240g skinless chicken
  breast fillet, sliced into 1cm
  strips
1 tsp turmeric
juice of 1 lemon
1 tbsp coconut oil
2 spring onions, cut into 1cm
  pieces
1 clove garlic, finely chopped
1 red chilli, de-seeded and
  finely chopped
1½ tbsp unsweetened peanut
  butter
2 handfuls of baby spinach
  leaves
½ tbsp light soy sauce
1 tsp sesame oil

Turmeric is packed with antioxidants and has powerful anti-inflammatory effects. This recipe is not only really good for you, but it also tastes delicious and works well for a lunch on the go.

METHOD

Chuck the chicken into a bowl, sprinkle over the turmeric and squeeze in the lemon juice. Mix the whole lot together with a metal spoon and let it sit for a couple of minutes.

Melt half of the coconut oil in a frying pan over a medium to high heat. Add the spring onions, garlic and chilli and stir-fry for about 2 minutes. Reduce the heat and pour in 50ml of water, quickly followed by the peanut butter.

Gently work the peanut butter into the liquid until it is fully combined. Drop in the spinach and stir over a medium heat until the leaves are wilted. Take the pan off the heat and stir in both the soy sauce and sesame oil. Leave the spinach satay to one side.

Melt the remaining coconut oil in a second pan over a high heat and scrape in the turmeric-stained chicken. Stir-fry for about 4 minutes, or until you are happy the chicken is fully cooked. Check by slicing into one of the larger pieces to make sure the meat is white all the way through, with no raw pink bits left.

Serve up the delicious chicken on top of the spinach satay sauce.

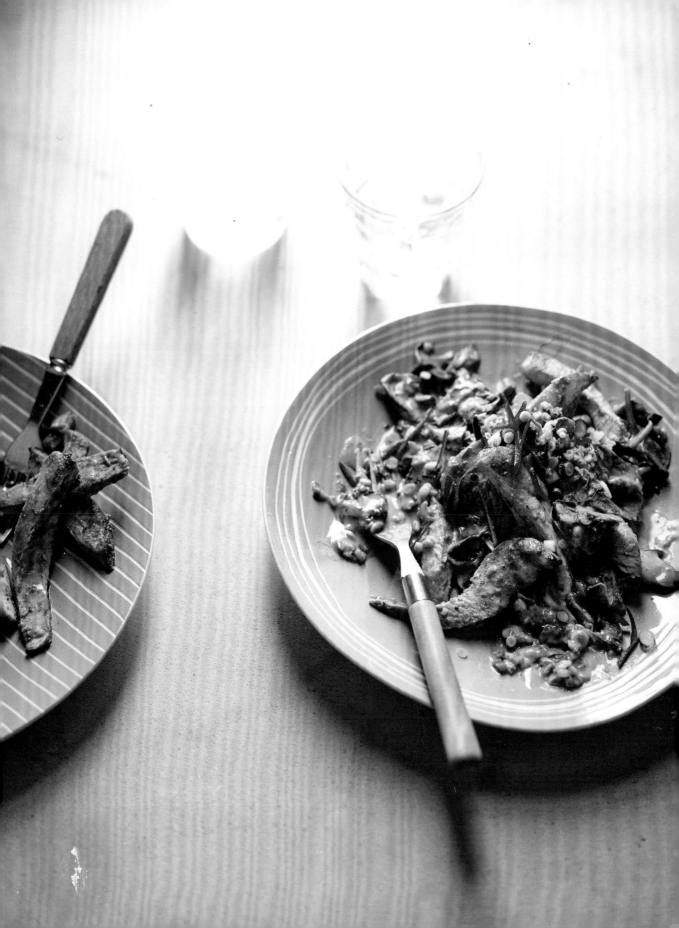

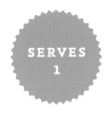

REDUCED-CARB
MAKE AHEAD
INGREDIENTS

1 tsp butter

5 chestnut mushrooms,
  roughly chopped

1 clove garlic, chopped

3 spring onions, finely sliced

1 x 240g skinless chicken
  breast fillet, sliced into 1cm
  strips

50ml chicken stock

2 large handfuls of watercress

salt and pepper

75ml double cream

2 tsp wholegrain mustard

15g parmesan, grated

CREAMY CHICKEN WITH MUSHROOMS

This is a fabulously rich-tasting recipe with a load of flavours you'll love. It's so easy to make and will be great the next day too, so it's ideal for a boss prep session.

METHOD

Melt the butter in a large frying pan over a medium to high heat. When bubbling, chuck in the mushrooms, garlic and spring onions and stir-fry for 2 minutes.

Slide in the chicken and continue to stir-fry everything together for about 4 minutes, by which time the mushrooms and chicken should have taken on a little colour. Check the chicken is cooked by slicing into one of the larger pieces to make sure the meat is white all the way through, with no raw pink bits left.

Pour in the chicken stock and bring to the boil. Get the watercress in there – a bit like spinach, it will wilt down, so don't be afraid to pile it high and watch it quickly shrink.

When the watercress has wilted, sprinkle in a pinch of salt and pepper and pour in the cream. Let the whole lot come back to the boil one last time and then stir in the mustard and parmesan just before serving up.

Delish.

SALMON AND PRAWNS WITH PARMESAN SAUCE

This recipe is ideal for when you want something warm and comforting on a rest day. You could also substitute chicken breast, if you're not into fish.

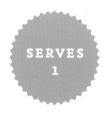

REDUCED-CARB INGREDIENTS

1 tsp butter

2 rashers of smoked back bacon, sliced into 1cm strips

¼ leek, trimmed, washed and finely shredded

5 midget trees (tender-stem broccoli), any bigger stalks sliced in half lengthways

1 x 190g skinless salmon fillet, chopped into large chunks

5 raw prawns, peeled and cleaned

100ml double cream

juice of ½ lemon

15g parmesan, grated

handful of parsley, roughly chopped

METHOD

Melt the butter in a large frying pan over a medium to high heat. When bubbling, chuck in the bacon, leek and midget trees and stir-fry for about 3 minutes, until the leek has softened and the bacon is pretty much cooked through.

Crank up the heat to maximum and get ready as the next bit doesn't take very long.

Add the salmon and prawns and toss with the other ingredients for about 1 minute, by which time the prawns should be turning from raw-grey to pink, which shows you they are cooked. Pour in about 30ml of water and let it steam up.

Quickly follow the water with the double cream and reduce the heat to medium. Let the cream bubble up and simmer away for 2 minutes to ensure the fish and prawns are totally cooked through.

When you are happy the seafood is fully cooked, squeeze in the lemon juice and stir in the parmesan and parsley.

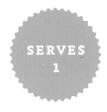

REDUCED-CARB
MAKE AHEAD
INGREDIENTS

2 eggs
½ tbsp coconut oil
1 x 125g skinless chicken
  breast, sliced into 1cm strips
2 tbsp mayonnaise
2 jarred anchovies, drained
  and roughly chopped
½ clove garlic, roughly
  chopped
10g parmesan, grated
¼ cucumber, de-seeded,
  halved and sliced
5 radishes, sliced
1 baby gem lettuce, leaves
  separated
15g pine nuts

CHEAT'S CHICKEN CAESAR

Forget about buying expensive lunches on the go. If you want to prep like a boss for work then give this one a try. It's so quick and easy to make and tastes great hot or cold.

METHOD

Bring a saucepan of water to the boil, then gently lower in the eggs and boil for 8 minutes for yolks that are still just soft. Remove from the pan and run under cold water before peeling.

While the eggs are cooking, melt the coconut oil in a large frying pan over a high heat. Slide in the chicken strips and fry for about 8 minutes, or until totally cooked through. Check by slicing into one of the larger pieces to make sure the meat is white all the way through, with no raw pink bits left.

Place the mayonnaise, anchovies, garlic, parmesan and 3 tablespoons of warm water in a small blender and blitz until you have a smooth dressing.

To serve, pile up all the fresh veg on your plate and top with the cooked chicken. Slice the eggs in half and place on top of the chicken. Drizzle with the dressing and scatter the whole lot with pine nuts.

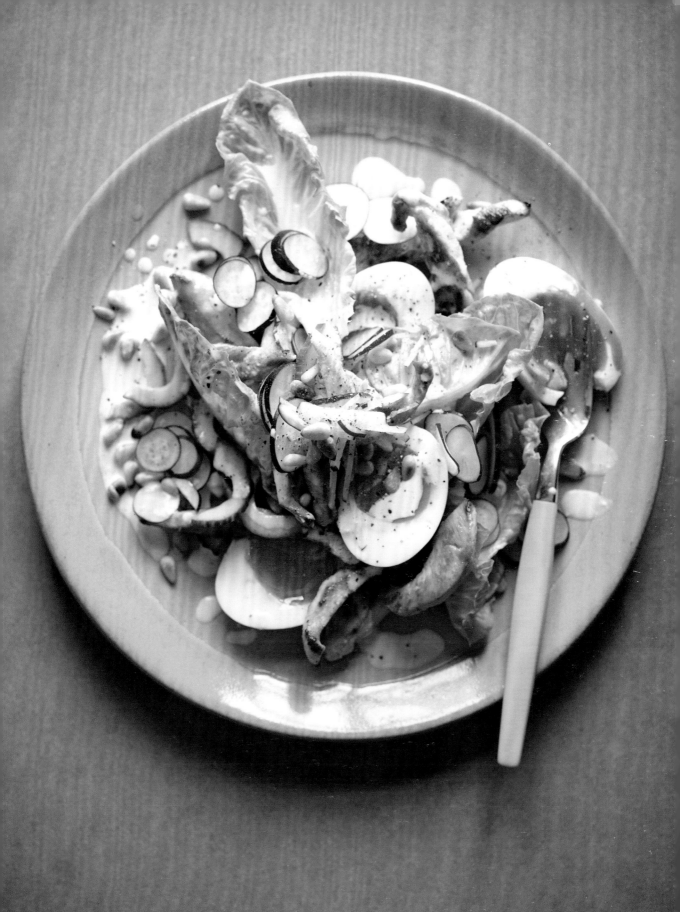

SEA BASS WITH PAK CHOI AND CASHEW NUTS

REDUCED-CARB INGREDIENTS

2 x 125g sea bass fillets,
 skin on
2 tsp olive oil
salt
½ tbsp coconut oil
2 pak choi, quartered
 lengthways
2 spring onions, finely sliced
1 clove garlic, finely sliced
40g cashew nuts
1 tbsp light soy sauce
1 tsp sesame seeds
1 red chilli, de-seeded and
 finely sliced, to serve –
 optional

So much of the goodness of sea bass is in the skin, so don't throw it away. It tastes best when it's crispy so give it a good grilling. The sesame seeds, cashews and olive oil give this dish plenty of healthy fats to fuel your body.

METHOD

Preheat your grill to maximum. Lay the fish fillets on a baking tray lined with baking parchment, drizzle with the olive oil and season with a little salt.

Grill the fillets for about 7 minutes on the skin side. The skin should crisp up and blister in spots. Flip the fillets and give them another minute. Make sure the fish is cooked by checking that the flesh has turned from a raw pale colour to cooked bright white, then turn off the grill and leave the fillets to keep warm until you're ready to eat.

While the fish is cooking, melt the coconut oil in a large frying pan or wok over a high heat. Chuck in the pak choi and stir-fry for 30 seconds. Quickly add the spring onions and garlic and stir-fry for a further minute.

Take the pan off the heat and carefully pour in 2 tablespoons of water – it will spit and bubble so watch out. When the pan has calmed down, slide it back over the heat and keep stir-frying for another 2 minutes until the water has pretty much evaporated.

Add the cashew nuts and toss to mix with the other ingredients, then remove the pan from the heat and stir through the light soy sauce and the sesame seeds.

Dish up the tasty veg and top with the grilled sea bass and chilli, if using, for an extra kick.

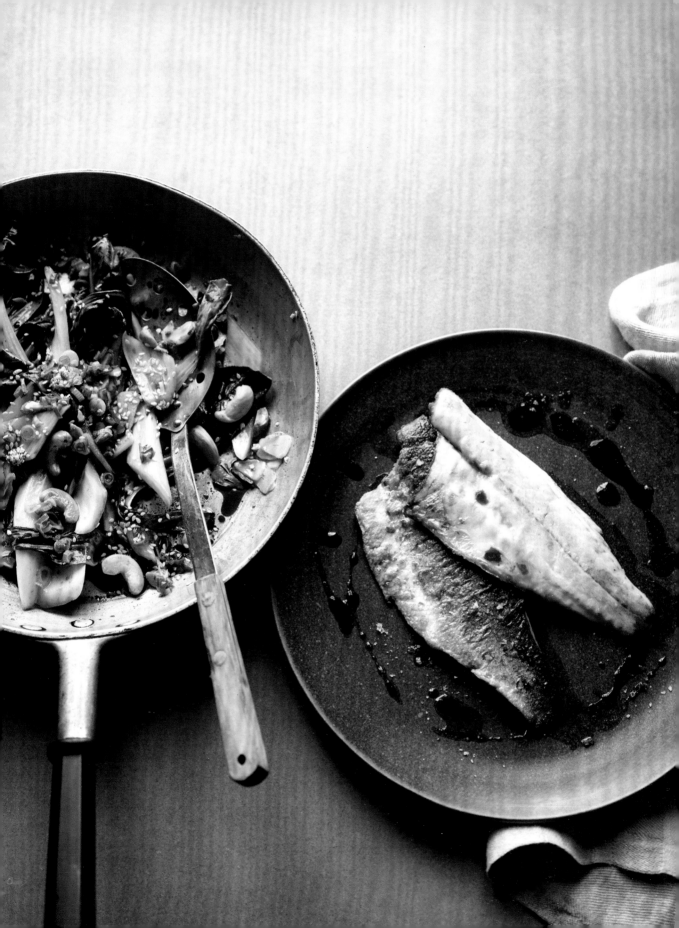

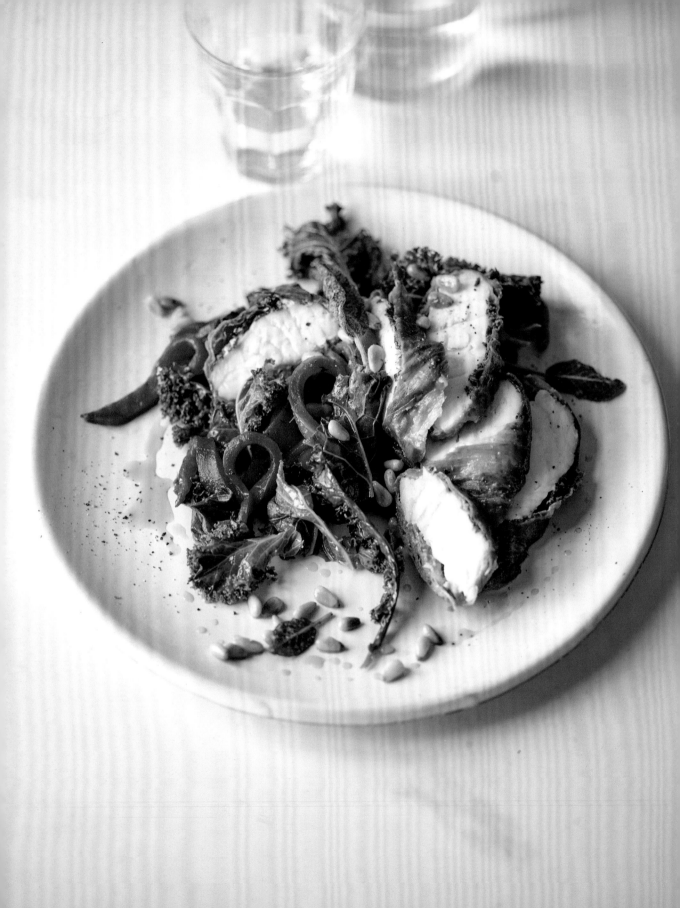

MONKFISH WRAPPED IN PARMA HAM

SERVES 1

REDUCED-CARB INGREDIENTS

4 slices of parma ham
1 x 225g monkfish fillet, trimmed
salt and pepper
5 sage leaves, finely chopped
1 tsp butter
1 jarred red pepper, drained and thinly sliced
20g pine nuts
large handful of kale, to serve

In my opinion, anything wrapped in parma ham is a winner! This will make a great sharing starter if you have a friend coming over for dinner.

METHOD

Put a saucepan of water on to boil.

Lay the parma ham slices side by side, with a slight overlap. Try to make the overall width of the ham roughly the same size as the length of the fish fillet.

Season the monkfish with a little salt and pepper and then sprinkle all over with the chopped sage. Place the fish along one end of the ham slices and then roll it up in the ham.

Melt the butter in a frying pan over a medium to high heat. When bubbling, carefully lay in the fish. Cook for about 2 minutes on each side and then add the red pepper slices and pine nuts. Continue cooking for a further minute or so, by which time the fish should be firm and the ham crispy.

Drop the kale into the water and simmer for about 2 minutes, or until tender, then drain in a sieve or colander.

Serve up the fish, scooping up all the red pepper slices and pine nuts, with a healthy side of steamed kale.

CHICKEN WITH CAULIFLOWER CHEESE

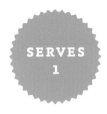

SERVES 1

REDUCED-CARB INGREDIENTS

⅓ cauliflower, florets only (about 200g)
1 tsp butter
½ onion, diced
6 sage leaves, finely sliced
1 x 200g skinless chicken breast fillet, sliced into 1cm strips
2 tbsp crème fraiche
1 egg yolk
10g parmesan, grated
50g cheddar, grated

I don't know why, but people always seem to go mad for cheesy Lean in 15 recipes. The flavours in this dish will remind you of a Sunday roast.

METHOD

Bring a saucepan of water to the boil and preheat your grill to maximum. When the water is boiling, chuck in the cauliflower florets and cook for 6 minutes.

Meanwhile, melt the butter in a frying pan over a medium to high heat. When bubbling, add the onion and cook, stirring regularly, for about 4 minutes, or until it's beginning to soften and turn translucent.

Crank up the heat and slide in the sage leaves and chicken and stir-fry for about 8 minutes, or until you are sure the chicken is cooked through. Check by slicing into one of the larger pieces to make sure the meat is white all the way through, with no raw pink bits left.

At the end of its cooking time, the cauliflower should be tender but still retain a bite. Drain the florets in a colander and then tumble them into a small baking dish. Whisk up the crème fraiche, egg yolk and both grated cheeses. Pour the cheesy mixture over the cauliflower and slide the dish under the grill, then leave it for about 4 minutes, or until bubbling and golden.

Serve up the cauliflower cheese scattered with the sage and onion chicken. This dish won't win prizes for its looks, but that's not going to bother you once you've tasted it.

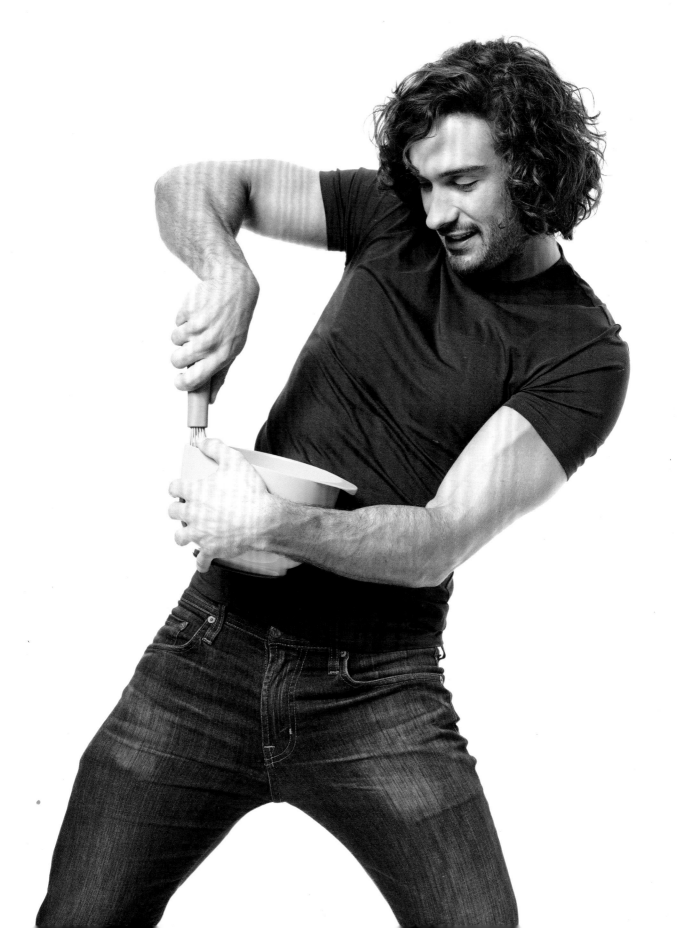

BASHED PORK WITH RED PEPPER MAYO

REDUCED-CARB INGREDIENTS

2 x 120g pork tenderloins
1 tsp butter
salt and pepper
1 sprig of rosemary, leaves
  only, finely chopped
2 sage leaves, finely sliced
30g mayonnaise
2 jarred red peppers, drained
  and roughly chopped
½ clove garlic, roughly
  chopped
big handful of rocket
20g whole almonds
juice of ½ lemon, to serve

Pork tenderloin can sometimes be a bit dry, but not when you cook it in butter and add this amazing red pepper mayo. I think you'll be pleasantly surprised when you try this one.

METHOD

Place the pork between two pieces of cling film or baking parchment on a chopping board. Using a rolling pin, meat mallet or any other blunt instrument, bash the meat until each piece is about 1cm thick. Make sure the loin is turned cut side up so you're bashing down into the grain.

Melt the butter in a large frying pan over a medium heat. Season the pork with salt and pepper and, when the butter is bubbling, add the herbs and cook for a few seconds, then gently lay the pork steaks in the pan. Fry for about 3 minutes on each side, or until cooked through – you can check this by slicing into a thick part of the meat to make sure there is no pink left.

While the pork is cooking, place the mayonnaise, red peppers and garlic in a small blender and blitz until smooth.

When the pork is cooked, remove to a plate and dab with a little kitchen roll to remove some of the fat. Arrange the steaks on your plate, top with the rocket and almonds and then drizzle over the mayonnaise.

Serve up with a sunny smile and a squeeze of lemon.

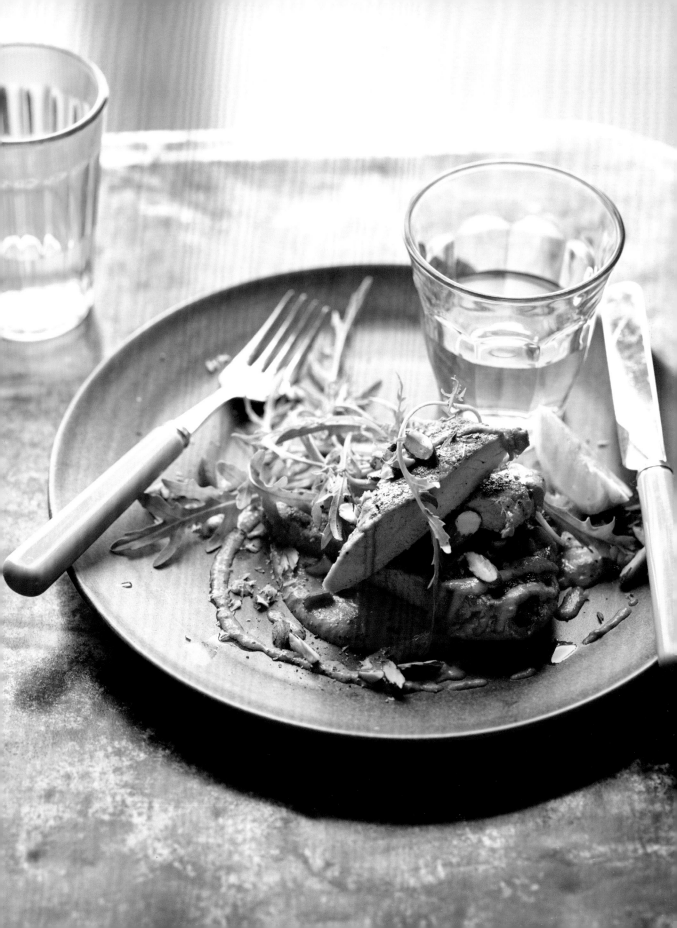

CHICKEN CAPRESE

Everybody knows the classic salad combination of mozzarella, tomatoes and basil. Well, this is my version, which kicks caprese's ass because I add chicken (like a boss!). If you fancy a change you could use another cheese, such as feta, and grill it in the oven so it goes all gooey.

METHOD

Melt the coconut oil in a frying pan over a medium to high heat. Add the chicken and stir-fry for about 6 minutes, or until you are happy the chicken is fully cooked. Check by slicing into one of the larger pieces to make sure the meat is white all the way through, with no raw pink bits left.

While the chicken is cooking, arrange your tomato slices, mozzarella slices and basil in an overlapping circle. Season with a little salt and pepper, and drizzle with the olive oil.

When you're ready to eat, top with the chicken, drizzle with the balsamic vinegar, scatter over the pine nuts, if using, and enjoy.

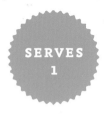

**SERVES
1**

REDUCED-CARB INGREDIENTS

½ tbsp coconut oil

1 x 240g skinless chicken breast fillet, sliced into 1cm strips

1 large tomato, cut into about 6 slices

1 x 125g ball of mozzarella, drained and cut into 6 slices

6 basil leaves, plus a few extra to garnish

salt and pepper

2 tsp olive oil

1 tbsp balsamic vinegar

20g pine nuts – optional

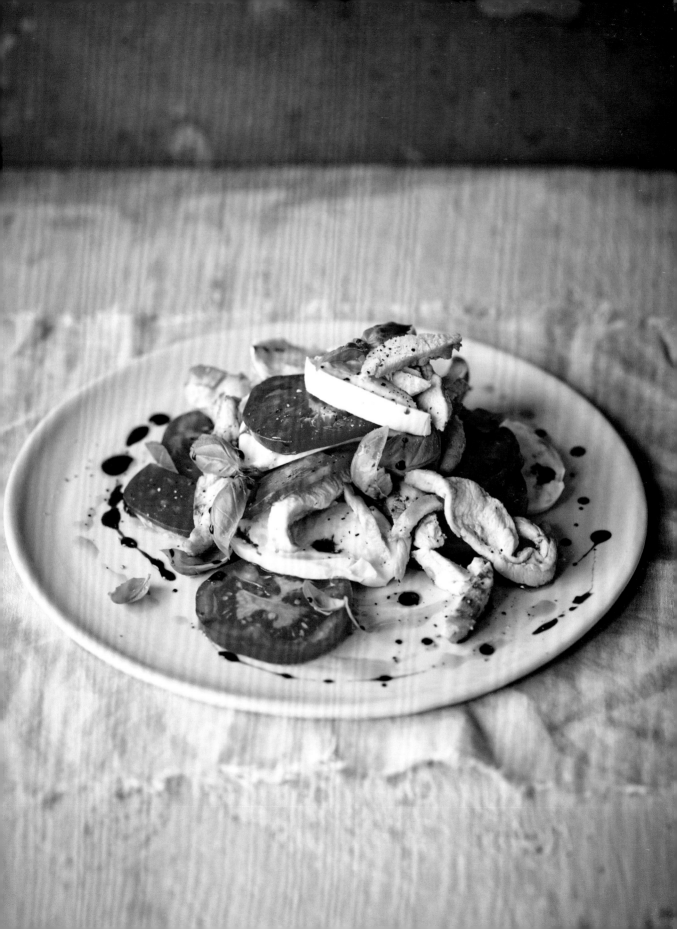

CAULIFLOWER RICE WITH COCONUT PRAWNS

SERVES 1

MAKE AHEAD

INGREDIENTS

1 tbsp coconut oil

3 spring onions, finely sliced

2 cloves garlic, finely chopped

3cm ginger, finely chopped

1 green chilli, de-seeded and
  finely chopped

3 tsp curry powder

1 tsp turmeric

200ml coconut milk

225g raw king prawns, peeled

40g mange tout or green
  beans

½ cauliflower, florets only
  (about 150g)

bunch of coriander, roughly
  chopped

juice of 1 lime

salt

Whoever came up with the idea for cauliflower rice is an absolute genius. Of course, there's no denying real rice is more satisfying, but the cauliflower alternative really does taste great and makes this the perfect low-carb dish without leaving you feeling hungry.

METHOD

Melt half of the coconut oil in a frying pan over a medium to high heat. Add the spring onions, garlic, ginger and chilli and stir-fry for 2 minutes. Sprinkle in the curry powder and turmeric and toss together with the other ingredients over the heat.

Pour in the coconut milk, crank up the heat and simmer for 2 minutes. Add the prawns and mange tout or green beans, bring the liquid back to the boil and simmer for about 1 minute before turning off the heat. Leave the prawns to cook in the residual heat.

Blitz the cauliflower florets in a food processor until they resemble small grains of rice or even couscous.

Melt the remaining coconut oil in another frying pan over a high heat. Scrape in the cauliflower and fry, stirring regularly, for about 3 minutes.

While the cauliflower is cooking, check the prawns are done – they should be coral pink all the way through. Do not be tempted to re-boil as you will ruin the precious prawns.

Stir the coriander and lime juice through the curry. Season the cauliflower with salt, slide into a bowl and serve alongside your tasty curry.

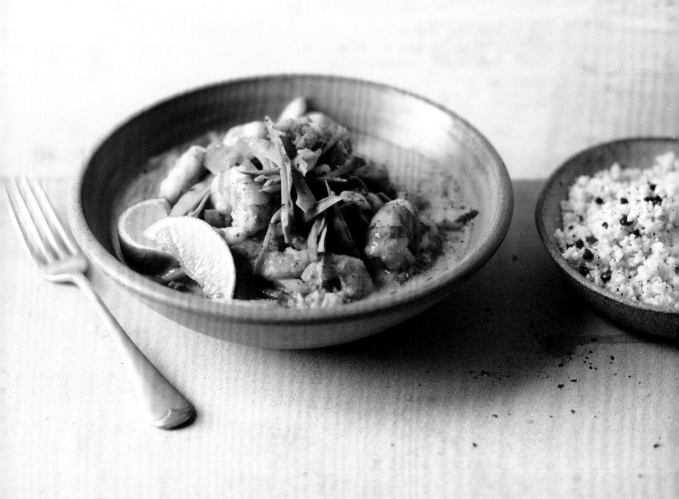

CHEESY CHICKEN WITH GARLIC AND CHIVES

SERVES 1

I'm sorry but anything with butter and mascarpone cheese is getting my vote. When I first made this absolute belter I was like, 'That recipe is going in my next book' – and here it is. Trust me, make it and you'll see why I had to include it #Creamer.

REDUCED-CARB INGREDIENTS

1 tsp butter
large handful of kale, stalks removed
2 cloves garlic, finely chopped
1 x 240g skinless chicken breast fillet, sliced into 1cm strips
¼ courgette, sliced into 5mm half-moons
30g mascarpone
10g grated parmesan
handful of chives, finely chopped
handful of parsley, roughly chopped
juice of 1 lemon

METHOD

Melt the butter in a large frying pan over a medium heat. When bubbling, drop in the kale and cook for about 4 minutes, stirring regularly. The kale should break down and become nice and tender.

Crank up the heat and add the garlic, chicken and courgette. Stir-fry for about 4 minutes, by which time the chicken should be pretty much cooked through and all the veg tender. Check the chicken is cooked by slicing into one of the larger pieces to make sure the meat is white all the way through, with no raw pink bits left.

Pour in about 2 tablespoons of water and reduce the heat to medium. Dollop in the mascarpone and, using a wooden spoon, stir gently as it melts. When the mascarpone has become a creamy sauce, bring it back up to the boil one last time and stir in the grated parmesan.

Remove the pan from the heat and stir through the chopped herbs before serving up with a good squeeze of lemon juice.

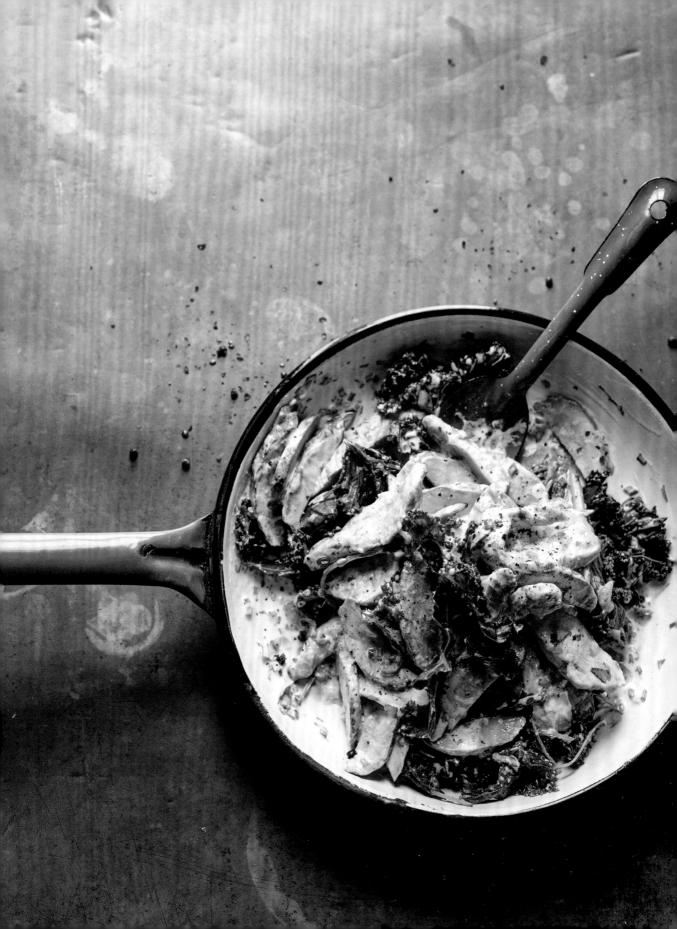

SAMMY SEA BASS WITH CRUNCHY CARROTS

**SERVES
1**

Oh, here he is. It's Sammy the sea bass showing his face again. He popped up in my previous books and he's back in this even tastier combo. This has got more healthy fats than you can shake a stick at. Go get lean.

REDUCED-CARB INGREDIENTS

2 x 125g sea bass fillets,
  skin on
drizzle of olive oil
salt
1 carrot, sliced into ribbons
½ cucumber, sliced into
  ribbons
3 radishes, sliced
1 red chilli, de-seeded and
  finely sliced
1 tbsp fish sauce
2 tsp sesame oil
juice of 1 lime
handful of coriander sprigs
35g cashew nuts, chopped

METHOD

Preheat your grill to maximum.

Lay the sea bass skin side up on a baking tray lined with baking parchment and drizzle with a little olive oil. Season the fish with salt and slide under the hot grill.

Cook the fish without turning for about 7 minutes, by which time the skin will have crisped up and blistered in a few places. Make sure the sea bass is done by checking that the flesh has turned from a raw pale colour to cooked bright white, then switch off the grill and leave the fillets to keep warm until you're ready to eat.

While the fish is grilling, put the carrot into a bowl with the cucumber, radishes and chilli. Pour over the fish sauce, sesame oil and lime juice and mix the whole lot together until all the ingredients are coated.

Plate up the carrot salad, slide on the sea bass, scatter over some coriander and finish off with the cashew nuts.

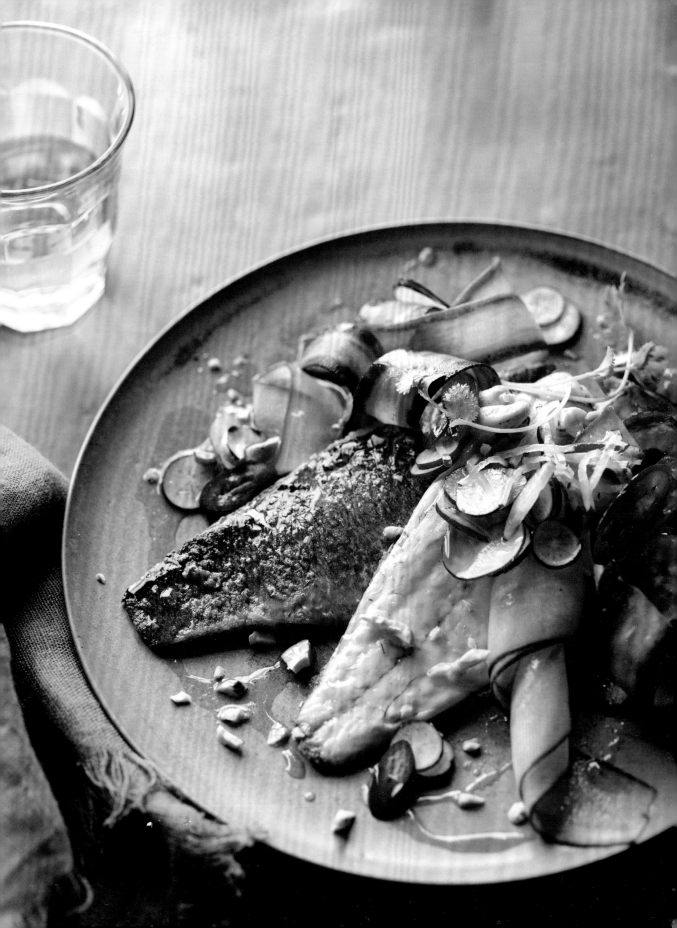

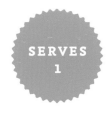

SERVES 1

INGREDIENTS

1 x 240g skinless chicken
  breast fillet, sliced into 1cm
  strips
juice of ½ lemon
½ tbsp smoked paprika
½ red onion, diced
2 cloves garlic, roughly
  chopped
3cm ginger, roughly chopped
1 red chilli, de-seeded and
  roughly chopped
1 tbsp tomato puree
½ tbsp coconut oil
½ tbsp garam masala
2 tsp turmeric
100ml coconut milk
25g ground almonds
handful of coriander, roughly
  chopped

CHICKEN TIKKA MASALA

Everyone loves a good curry, right? This one is legit. Homemade, healthy and Lean in 15. This recipe is perfect for cooking up in big batches, so get your mates round and have a curry night.

METHOD

Plonk the chicken into a bowl, add the lemon juice and smoked paprika, then give it all a good stir to make sure the chicken is well coated.

Chuck the onion, garlic, ginger, chilli and tomato puree into a blender with about 2 tablespoons of warm water and blitz until the ingredients are smooth.

Melt the coconut oil in a large frying pan over a medium to high heat. Scrape in the blitzed onion mixture and fry, stirring almost constantly, for 2 minutes. Next add the marinated chicken to the pan and continue stir-frying for another 2 minutes.

Sprinkle in the garam masala and turmeric and stir to mix. Pour in the coconut milk and bring up to the boil. Simmer for about 5 minutes, or until you are certain the chicken is cooked through. Check by slicing into one of the larger pieces to make sure the meat is white all the way through, with no raw pink bits left.

Remove the pan from the heat and stir in the ground almonds and coriander. Scoop onto a plate and get stuck right in.

PORK CHOP WITH CREAMY GREENS

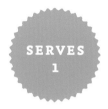

SERVES 1

REDUCED-CARB INGREDIENTS

1 large pork chop (about 275g), trimmed of most fat
salt and pepper
1 tsp butter
½ onion, diced
2 cloves garlic, finely chopped
100g spring greens, stalks removed
50g kale, stalks removed
50ml chicken stock
50ml double cream
2 tsp Dijon mustard
juice of ½ lemon
25g walnuts, roughly chopped

This is another really simple recipe to make and the creamy greens bring the pork chop to life. You could also try this with chicken if you fancy a change.

METHOD

Preheat your grill to maximum and put a saucepan of water on to boil.

Place the chop on the grill pan, season with salt and pepper and slide under the grill. Cook for about 7 minutes on each side, or until you are happy the chop is cooked through – you can check this by cutting into one of the thicker parts to make sure there is no pink left.

While the chop is grilling, melt the butter in a large frying pan over a medium heat. When bubbling, chuck in the onion and garlic and fry gently for about 3 minutes.

When the water is boiling, drop in the spring greens and kale and boil for about 45 seconds, then drain in a sieve or colander. Rinse under cold running water to cool the leaves down, then give them a good shake to remove as much of the excess liquid as possible.

Dump the leaves into the pan with the onions and garlic and stir before pouring in the stock and cream. Bring to the boil and simmer for about 1 minute. Stir in the mustard and lemon juice, season with a little salt and pepper and then remove the sauce from the heat.

Lay the pork on a plate, spoon over the tasty greens and finish with a scattering of chopped walnuts.

CHICKEN KIEV WITH CAULIFLOWER RICE

REDUCED-CARB INGREDIENTS

1 x 240g skinless chicken
   breast fillet
salt and pepper
25g softened butter, plus a
   small knob
⅓ cauliflower, florets only
   (about 200g)
½ tbsp coconut oil
1 large clove garlic, minced
   or crushed
small handful of parsley,
   roughly chopped
15g roughly chopped walnuts
green salad, to serve

I love turning typically un-lean meals into lean ones.
This chicken kiev uses walnuts instead of breadcrumbs,
so it's reduced-carb but contains healthy fats. The
garlic butter is incredible with the cauliflower rice, too.

METHOD

Place the chicken between two pieces of cling film or baking
parchment on a chopping board. Using a rolling pin, meat
mallet or any other blunt instrument, bash the chicken until
it is about 1cm thick all over. Season with a little salt and pepper.

Melt the knob of butter in a frying pan over a medium to
high heat. When bubbling, carefully lay in the chicken breast.
Cook for about 4 minutes on each side, or until you are
certain it is cooked through. Check by slicing into a thicker
part to make sure the meat is white all the way through, with
no raw pink bits left.

Meanwhile, blitz the cauliflower florets in a food processor
until they resemble small grains of rice or even couscous.

Melt the coconut oil in a second pan over a high heat. Add
the cauliflower and fry, stirring regularly, for about 4 minutes.

Beat the softened butter together with the garlic and most
of the chopped parsley until well combined. Then spoon the
garlic butter into the pan with the chicken. As the butter melts
and the garlic cooks a little, turn the breast over a few times
to get maximum garlic coverage. Cook the chicken in the butter
for 1 minute.

Serve up the cauliflower rice and top with the chicken breast.
Spoon over the garlic butter and chopped walnuts, sprinkle
with the remaining parsley and serve with a side salad.

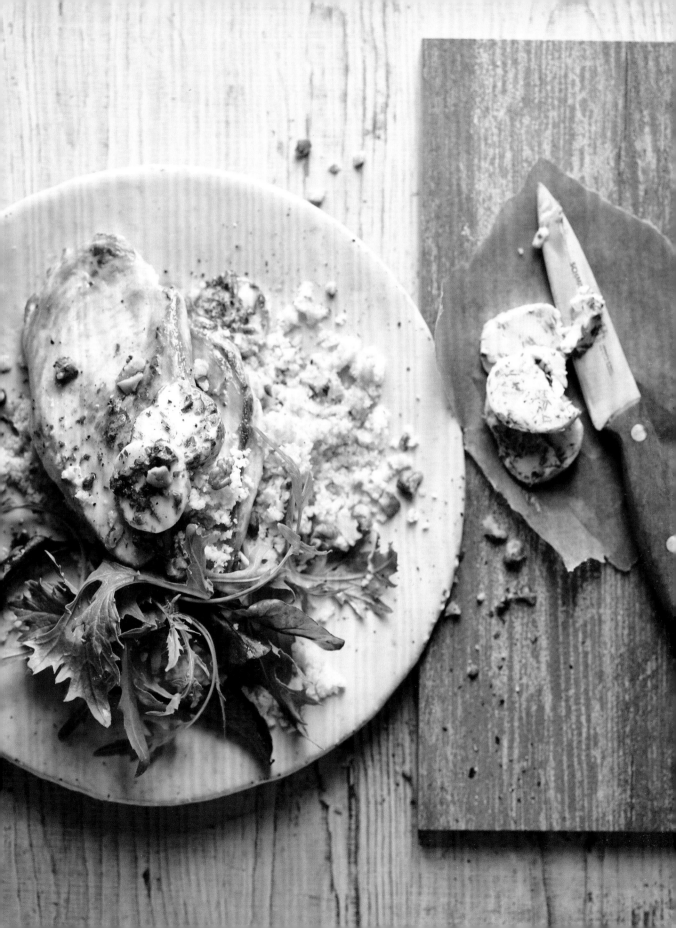

CAJUN SALMON WITH SWEETCORN AND CUCUMBER RELISH

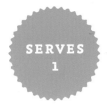

SERVES 1

Cajun is one of those spice mixes that goes well with everything. The healthy fats from the salmon, avocado and nuts will give you energy for hours and hours.

REDUCED-CARB INGREDIENTS

1½ tbsp Cajun seasoning

2 tbsp olive oil

2 x 120g skinless salmon fillets

1 tbsp coconut oil

¼ cucumber, de-seeded and finely sliced

2 spring onions, finely sliced

110g tinned sweetcorn, drained

1 red chilli, de-seeded and finely sliced

3 cherry tomatoes, quartered

2 tsp red wine vinegar

handful of coriander, roughly chopped

salt and pepper

½ ripe avocado, de-stoned

15g cashew nuts, roughly chopped

lemon wedges, to serve

METHOD

Mix the Cajun seasoning with half of the olive oil and swoosh the salmon fillets to coat them.

Melt the coconut oil in a frying pan over a medium heat and gently lay in the salmon fillets. Cook the fish for about 8 minutes, turning regularly.

Meanwhile, chuck all the ingredients apart from the avocado, cashew nuts and lemon wedges into a bowl and season with salt and pepper. Scoop out large chunks of avocado straight into the relish before giving everything one last mix.

By now the salmon should be cooked through – you can check this by slicing into the thick end of a fillet to make sure the flesh has turned matt pink in colour.

Slide the salmon fillets onto a plate, top with the sweetcorn relish and finish with a scattering of cashew nuts. Serve with lemon wedges to squeeze over.

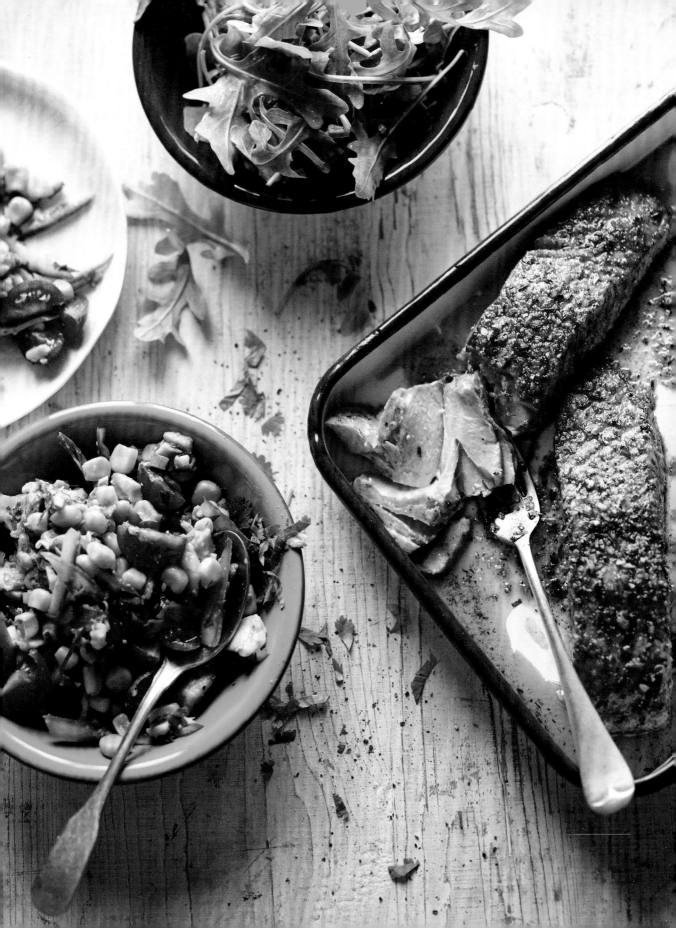

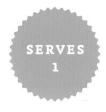

LAMB CUTLETS WITH COURGETTE AND SPINACH

If you've got a date coming over for dinner and want to impress them, then give this recipe a go. It's simple but tastes so good they will fall in love with you right there on the spot.

REDUCED-CARB INGREDIENTS

3 lamb cutlets
½ red onion, roughly chopped
2 cloves garlic, roughly chopped
3cm ginger, roughly chopped
1 tbsp coconut oil
¼ courgette, sliced into 5mm half-moons
1 green chilli, de-seeded and finely sliced
2 tsp garam masala
1 tomato, roughly chopped
2 large handfuls of baby spinach leaves
handful of coriander, roughly chopped

METHOD

Preheat your grill to maximum. Lay the lamb cutlets on a baking tray and grill them for about 5 minutes on one side and then 4 minutes on the other. When cooked, turn off the grill and leave the lamb to rest until you're ready to eat.

While the lamb is grilling, chuck the onion, garlic and ginger into a food processor and blitz until pretty much smooth.

Melt the coconut oil in a large frying pan over a high heat. Add the blitzed onion mixture and fry, stirring regularly, for 2 minutes. Add the courgette and chilli and stir-fry for a further 2 minutes, keeping the heat on high.

Sprinkle in the garam masala and stir to mix. Scrape in the chopped tomato and fry for 1 minute, or until it just starts to soften.

Reduce the heat a little and stir through the spinach until the leaves have wilted. Finish off by adding a good handful of chopped coriander.

Serve up the spiced spinach and top with the grilled lamb cutlets.

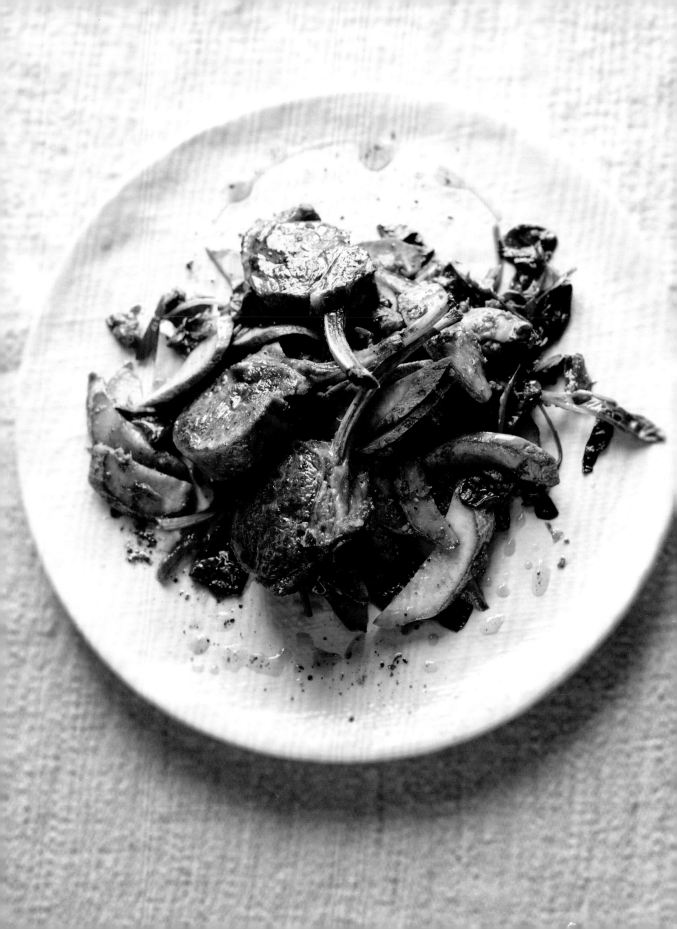

CHORIZO, CAVOLO NERO AND COD

SERVES 1

REDUCED-CARB INGREDIENTS

½ tbsp coconut oil
40g chorizo, roughly chopped into 1cm pieces
½ red onion, diced
100g cavolo nero, stalks removed
1 x 200g skinless cod fillet, chopped into 3cm chunks
5 cherry tomatoes, halved
1 tbsp tomato puree
25g cheddar
20g pine nuts
handful of parsley, roughly chopped

Sorry, but I can't get enough of chorizo – it makes everything taste so good! Is there anything it doesn't go well with? Cavolo nero is the new kale on the block and is jam-packed with healthy vitamins and minerals.

METHOD

Melt the coconut oil in a frying pan over a medium heat. Add the chorizo and onion and cook, stirring occasionally, for 2 minutes. Add the cavolo nero and cook for 1 minute, or until just beginning to wilt.

Crank up the heat to maximum and add the cod and tomatoes. Stir-fry for about 3 minutes, or until the fish is cooked through – you can check this by cutting into one of the thickest pieces to make sure it has turned from raw, pale flesh to cooked bright white.

Squeeze in the tomato puree and stir in. Pour in 50ml of water and reduce the heat to a slow bubble.

Scatter over the cheddar cheese and let it melt in the residual heat.

Finish the dish with the pine nuts and a generous sprinkling of chopped parsley.

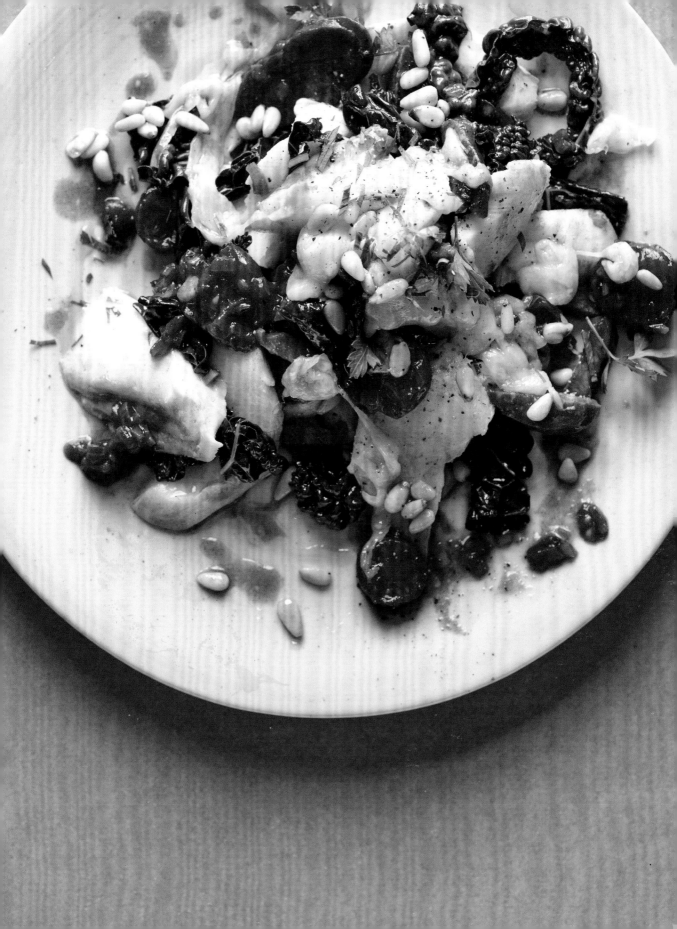

SALMON FILLET WITH WILD MUSHROOM SAUCE

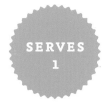

REDUCED-CARB INGREDIENTS

2 tsp butter
2 x 120g skinless salmon fillets
150g mixed wild mushrooms, chopped to roughly the same size
1 clove garlic, finely sliced
2 tbsp crème fraiche
large handful of baby spinach leaves
small handful each of chives and parsley, roughly chopped
30g cheddar, grated
juice of ½ lemon

Mushrooms are a love-them-or-hate-them kind of thing. These days you can find so many different types in the supermarket that it'd be a shame not to find one you like. A packet of mixed wild mushrooms gives you a good spread of tastes and textures.

METHOD

Melt half of the butter in a frying pan over a medium heat. When bubbling, carefully lay in the salmon fillets. Cook the fish for about 8 minutes, turning regularly.

While the fish is cooking, melt the remaining butter in another pan over a medium to high heat. When bubbling, chuck in the mushrooms and stir-fry for 2 minutes – try to get a little colour on them. Add the garlic and fry for 1 minute before pouring in 1 tablespoon of water and the crème fraiche. Work the crème fraiche in the pan until it melts, then reduce the heat a little so that the sauce is just simmering away.

Add the spinach and let it wilt into the creamy sauce. Sprinkle in the chopped herbs and the cheddar, again stirring everything together to help melt the cheese.

By now your fish should be cooked through – you can check this by slicing into the thick end of a fillet to make sure the flesh has turned matt pink in colour. Plate up the salmon and pour over the mushroom sauce.

Serve up with a squeeze of fresh lemon juice.

GARLICKY KALE WITH GRILLED CHICKEN

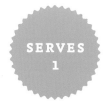

REDUCED-CARB INGREDIENTS

1 x skinless chicken breast
   fillet
1 tbsp coconut oil
salt and pepper
50g kale, stalks removed
1 clove garlic, finely chopped
60g oyster mushrooms, large
   ones ripped in half
2 spring onions, finely sliced
50ml chicken stock
75ml double cream
10g parmesan, grated
handful of parsley, roughly
   chopped
juice of ½ lemon

Kale can be a bit boring and bland, but not in this recipe, where it's combined with garlic and a naughty bit of double cream. I've gone with oyster mushrooms for a change here but you can use any type you prefer.

METHOD

Place the chicken between two pieces of cling film or baking parchment on a chopping board. Using a rolling pin, meat mallet or any other blunt instrument, bash the chicken until it is about 1cm thick all over.

Melt half of the coconut oil in a frying pan over a medium to high heat. Season the chicken with salt and pepper and gently lay in the pan. Fry for about 5 minutes on each side, by which time it will be pretty much cooked through.

While the chicken is cooking, melt the remaining coconut oil in a second pan, again over a medium to high heat. Chuck in the kale and cook, stirring regularly, for about 5 minutes, or until the leaves are wilting and almost tender.

Crank up the heat to maximum and add the garlic, mushrooms and spring onions and stir-fry for about 3 minutes, or until the mushrooms take on a little colour.

Now scoop up the chicken breast, nestle it in with the kale and mushrooms and pour in the chicken stock. Bring to the boil, then add the cream and bring to a simmer. The chicken will definitely be cooked by now, but if you're unsure just slice into a thicker part to make sure the meat is white all the way through, with no raw pink bits left.

Take the pan off the heat and stir through the parmesan, the parsley and the lemon juice.

MOROCCAN MONKFISH

SERVES 1

'Ras el hanout' may sound exotic but check out the spice aisle in your supermarket and you will be pleasantly surprised. The fish in this dish tastes incredible with the Moroccan spice blend and the flavours coming from the chorizo.

REDUCED-CARB INGREDIENTS

1 tbsp olive oil
3 tsp ras el hanout
2 x 120g monkfish fillets, trimmed and roughly chopped into 4cm chunks
30g chorizo, roughly chopped into 1cm pieces
3 spring onions, finely sliced
1 clove garlic, finely sliced
¼ red pepper, de-seeded and sliced into 1cm strips
5 cherry tomatoes, halved
1 tsp ground cumin
1 tbsp tomato puree
1 ripe avocado, sliced
20g pine nuts
handful of parsley, roughly chopped – optional

★ Serve with a pile of midget trees (tender-stem broccoli) and spinach or green beans.

METHOD

Pour half of the olive oil into a bowl and then sprinkle in the ras el hanout. Swish the monkfish about in the spiced oil until lightly coated.

Heat the remaining olive oil in a frying pan over a medium to high heat. Add the chorizo and fry on its own for about 1 minute. Next, add the spring onions, garlic, red pepper, cherry tomatoes and the monkfish, making sure you scrape out all of the oil and spice from the bowl.

Fry the whole lot together for about 3 minutes, then sprinkle in the cumin and squeeze in the tomato puree. Fry, stirring almost constantly, for 1 minute, and then stir in 100ml of water to make a sauce.

Put a lid on your pan and simmer for 1–2 minutes, or until you are sure the fish is fully cooked through – you can check this by slicing into one of the biggest chunks to make sure it has turned from raw, pale flesh to cooked bright white.

When you're happy the fish is cooked, tip it into a bowl and top with the avocado slices, pine nuts and parsley, if using.

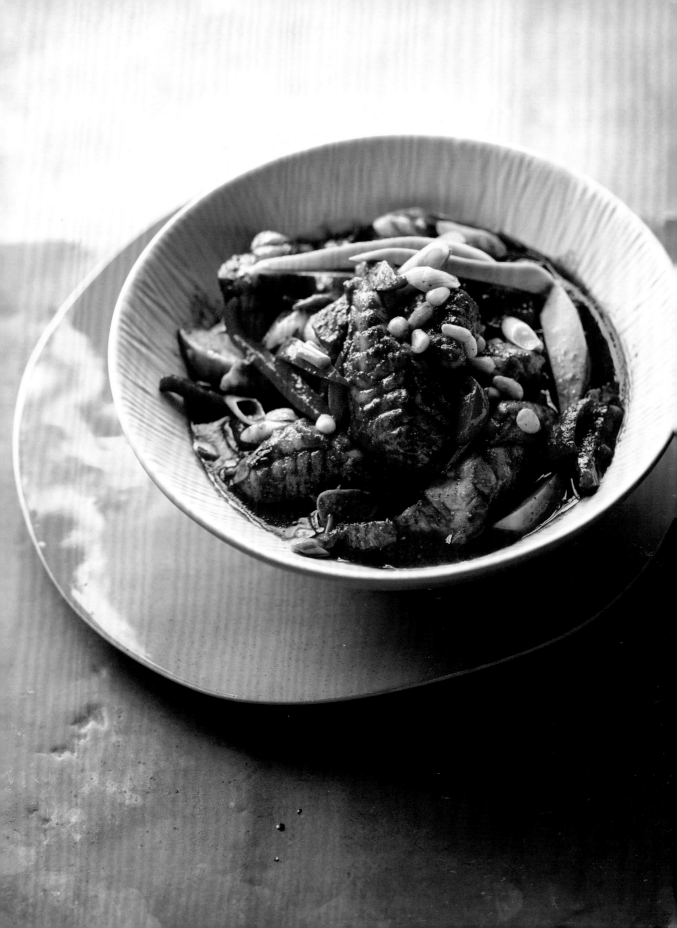

STRAIGHT-UP STEAK WITH BLUE MUSHROOMS

SERVES 1

REDUCED-CARB
INGREDIENTS

2 portobello mushrooms
1 x 240g sirloin steak
salt and pepper
20g blue cheese (I like to use
   Roquefort)
20g mascarpone
small handful of chives, finely
   chopped
4 cherry tomatoes on the vine
large handful of watercress,
   to serve

When I eat out, I love to order a good steak. I couldn't release a book without at least one steak recipe. This one with blue cheese is off the hook. You're going to love it. #SteakMe.

METHOD

Preheat a griddle pan over a high heat and preheat your grill to maximum.

Remove the mushroom stalks and discard. Season the steak and mushrooms with a little salt and pepper. When the griddle is hot, carefully lay the mushrooms skin side down in the pan, followed by the steak.

Cook the mushrooms for 2 minutes on one side only and remove. Cook the steak for 4 minutes on each side for medium rare. Transfer the steak to a plate and keep it warm until you're ready to eat.

While the steak is cooking, break the blue cheese into a bowl, dollop in the mascarpone and slide in the chives. Beat together until smooth, then spoon and press the mixture into the grilled side of the mushrooms. Place the mushrooms, cheese side up, on a baking tray with the tomatoes alongside. Grill the vegetables for about 6 minutes, or until the cheese has melted and is bubbling up.

It doesn't matter how you serve this one up – just get all the ingredients onto a plate, chuck on a handful of watercress to freshen things up, and get stuck in.

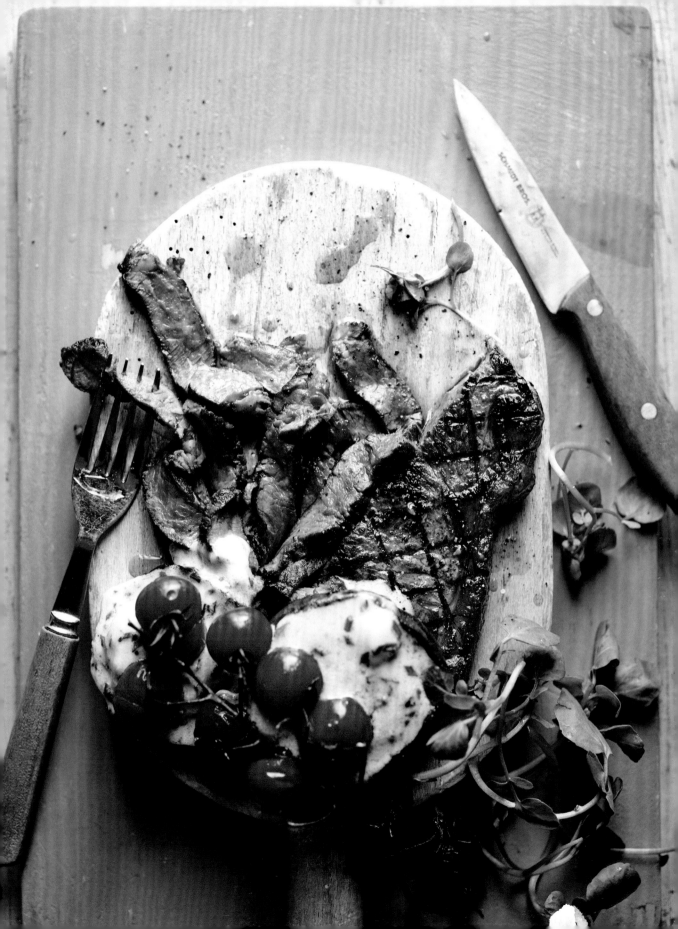

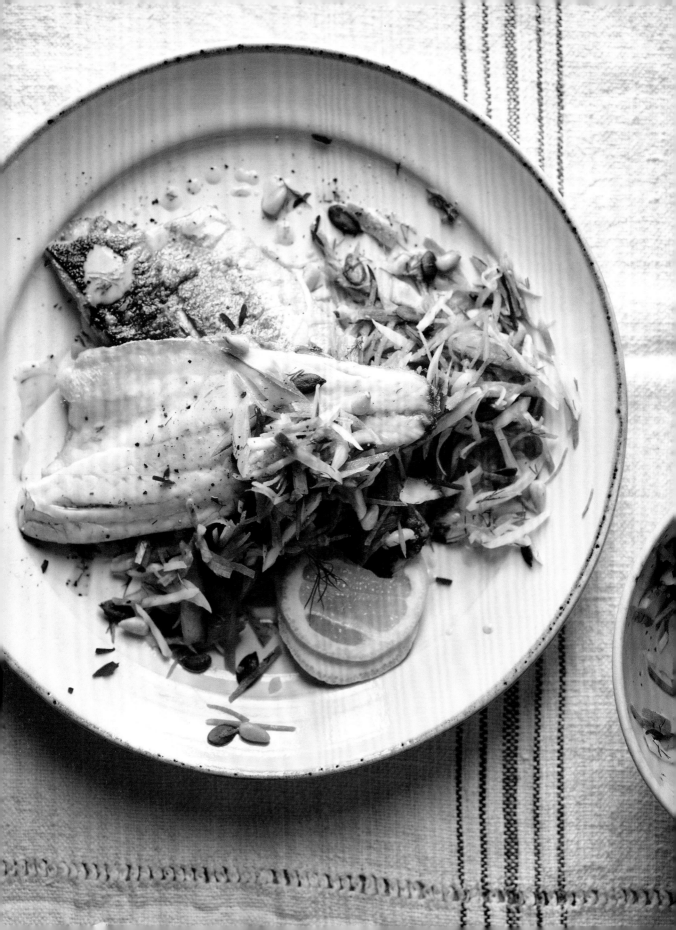

SEA BASS WITH LEMON AND FENNEL COLESLAW

If you're looking to impress friends at a dinner party then this grilled fish dish is just the ticket. The flavours from the dill and fennel bring it to life and will leave everyone wanting more.

REDUCED-CARB INGREDIENTS

2 x 120g sea bass fillets, skin on
2 tbsp olive oil
salt
½ fennel bulb, grated
¼ cucumber, de-seeded and grated
½ red chilli, de-seeded and finely sliced
½ carrot, grated
20g pine nuts
small handful of dill, leaves only, roughly chopped
20g pumpkin seeds
juice of ½ lemon, plus a couple of slices, to serve
1 tsp Dijon mustard

METHOD

Preheat your grill to maximum.

Lay the sea bass fillets, skin side up, on a grill pan lined with baking parchment and drizzle over half a tablespoon of the olive oil. Season the fillets with salt, then slide them under the grill and cook for 7 minutes without turning. Make sure the fish is cooked by checking that the flesh has turned from a raw pale colour to cooked bright white, then turn off the grill and leave the fillets to keep warm until you're ready to eat.

While the fish is cooking, toss together the fennel, cucumber, chilli, carrot, pine nuts, dill and pumpkin seeds in a large bowl.

Mix the remaining oil with the lemon juice and mustard until they become a smooth dressing. Pour over the vegetables and toss until well coated.

Serve up the coleslaw topped with the grilled sea bass fillets.

COD WITH CHEESY HERB SAUCE

REDUCED-CARB INGREDIENTS

75g cream cheese
20g cheddar, grated
1 tbsp chives, chopped
1 tbsp tarragon, chopped
1 spring onion, finely chopped
zest of ¼ lemon
salt and pepper
1 x 220g skinless cod fillet
1 chicken or fish stock cube
½ tbsp coconut oil
4 cherry tomatoes, halved
2 large handfuls of spinach
10g pine nuts

This is a great way to cook fish without drying it out as the stock bath helps to keep it nice and moist. If you fancy a change, feel free to swap the herbs for some others – mint and basil work really well too.

METHOD

Preheat your oven to 190°C (fan 170°C, gas mark 5) and put your kettle on to boil.

Dollop the cream cheese into a bowl and add the cheddar, chives, tarragon, spring onion, lemon zest and a good pinch of salt and pepper. Mix together well.

Lay the cod in a small baking dish and spread the cheesy mixture evenly over the fish – I find the back of a spoon works best for this.

Stir the stock cube into 500ml of the boiling water from the kettle and pour it carefully into the dish around the fish – do not pour it directly onto the cod! Slide the dish into the oven and bake for 10 minutes.

While the fish is cooking, melt the coconut oil in a large frying pan over a medium to high heat. When hot, add the cherry tomatoes and fry for 2 minutes until they are just starting to soften. Add the spinach and stir to wilt it. Season with a little more salt and pepper and remove the pan from the heat.

When you're happy that the fish is cooked through – check by cutting into it to make sure it has turned from raw, pale flesh to cooked bright white – remove the dish from the oven, spoon the vegetables onto a plate and lay the cod on top. Finish with a sprinkling of pine nuts.

BEEF AND BLACK OLIVE MEATBALLS

SERVES
1

REDUCED-CARB
GOOD TO FREEZE

INGREDIENTS

½ tbsp coconut oil
225g beef meatballs, about
  7, from a packet
½ red onion, diced
7 pitted black olives, roughly
  chopped
1 clove garlic, roughly chopped
½ red pepper, de-seeded and
  roughly chopped
15g grated parmesan
150g tinned chopped tomatoes
large handful of baby spinach
  leaves
½ ball of mozzarella (roughly
  75g)
20g pine nuts
handful of basil, roughly
  chopped

Juicy meatballs with a cheesy mozzarella sauce – how can food this delicious be good for you? Remember, healthy food can taste great too. Make this for the whole family and they will love you. This is a reduced-carb meal, though, so don't try to sneak in pasta or garlic bread.

METHOD

Melt the coconut oil in a large frying pan over a medium to high heat and roll in the meatballs until they have browned all over.

Meanwhile, put the onion, olives, garlic, red pepper, parmesan and tomatoes into a food processor and blitz until pretty much smooth.

When the meatballs are brown, tip the tomato mix into the pan and bring up to the boil. Simmer for 8–10 minutes, or until you are happy the meatballs are cooked through, then chuck in the spinach and gently stir it through the sauce until the leaves have wilted.

Finally, rip up the mozzarella and dot it about in the sauce. Give the whole lot 1 minute with a lid on and then spoon it triumphantly into a bowl.

Finish by scattering with pine nuts and chopped basil.

CHICKEN AND PARMESAN MELTS

Don't be a melt and skip this recipe. Trust me, you're going to love it. I mean, come on, just look at it. Melted cheese on fried chicken – how can you resist?

REDUCED-CARB INGREDIENTS

1 x 240g skinless chicken
  breast fillet
salt and pepper
1 tsp butter
150g tinned chopped tomatoes
5 pitted black olives, roughly
  halved
2 tsp dried Italian herbs
10g grated parmesan
40g mozzarella, grated
½ ripe avocado
large handful of baby spinach
  leaves, rocket or watercress,
  to serve

METHOD

Preheat your grill to maximum.

Place the chicken between two pieces of cling film or baking parchment on a chopping board. Using a rolling pin, meat mallet or any other blunt instrument, bash the chicken until it is about 1cm thick all over. Season with salt and pepper.

Melt the butter in a frying pan over a medium to high heat. When bubbling, gently slide in the bashed chicken and fry for about 4 minutes without turning.

While the chicken is frying, mix together the tomatoes, olives and dried herbs, and add a little salt and pepper.

Flip the chicken and then take it off the heat. Pile the tomato mix onto the fried side of the chicken and then sprinkle over the parmesan and mozzarella.

Slide the frying pan under the hot grill. If your pan has a plastic handle then be sure not to slide the pan in too far. Grill the chicken for about 4 minutes, or until the cheeses have melted and are bubbling. The chicken should be cooked through – check by slicing into a thicker part to make sure the meat is white all the way through, with no raw pink bits left.

Serve up the chicken melt with the avocado and a large portion of fresh salad greens.

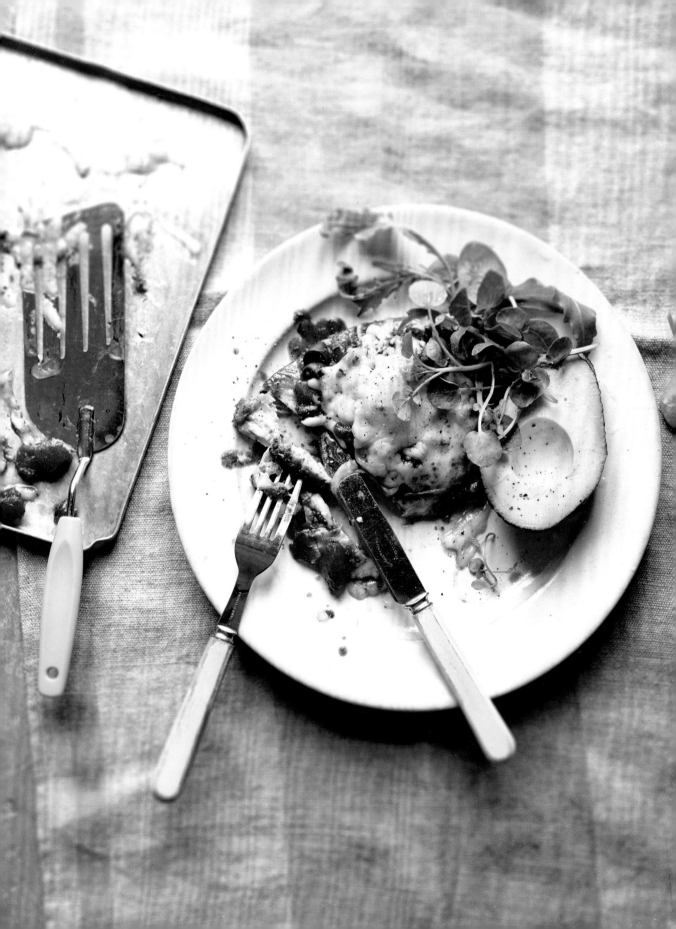

COURGETTI WITH MISO STEAK

SERVES
1

Everyone is loving spiralized veg these days, but if you don't have a spiralizer just run a peeler all the way down the length of the courgette to produce large ribbons, then slice those ribbons with a knife into thin strips. Takes a bit longer, but still just as tasty.

REDUCED-CARB INGREDIENTS

150g white miso paste
1 x 240g sirloin steak, trimmed
 of visible fat
½ tbsp coconut oil
1 clove garlic, sliced
4 cherry tomatoes, halved
1 courgette, topped and tailed
large handful of baby spinach
 leaves
25g pine nuts

METHOD

Preheat a griddle pan over a high heat.

Splodge the miso paste into a bowl and pour in about 3 tablespoons of warm water, or just enough to make the paste spreadable. Lay the steak in the miso and swoosh it around until well coated.

When the griddle pan is smoking hot, fry the steak for 4 minutes on each side for medium rare. When cooked, remove the steak to a plate to rest until you're ready to eat.

While the steak is cooking, melt the coconut oil in a frying pan over a medium heat. Chuck in the garlic and tomatoes and stir-fry gently for 1 minute, which is about enough time to put the courgette through the spiralizer.

When you have a pile of courgette, crank up the heat under the frying pan and tip it in with the garlic and tomatoes. Stir-fry everything together for about 1 minute and then add the spinach. When the spinach has wilted and the courgette has warmed through, take the pan off the heat and pile the cooked veg high on a plate. Lay your perfectly charred steak on top and scatter over the pine nuts to serve.

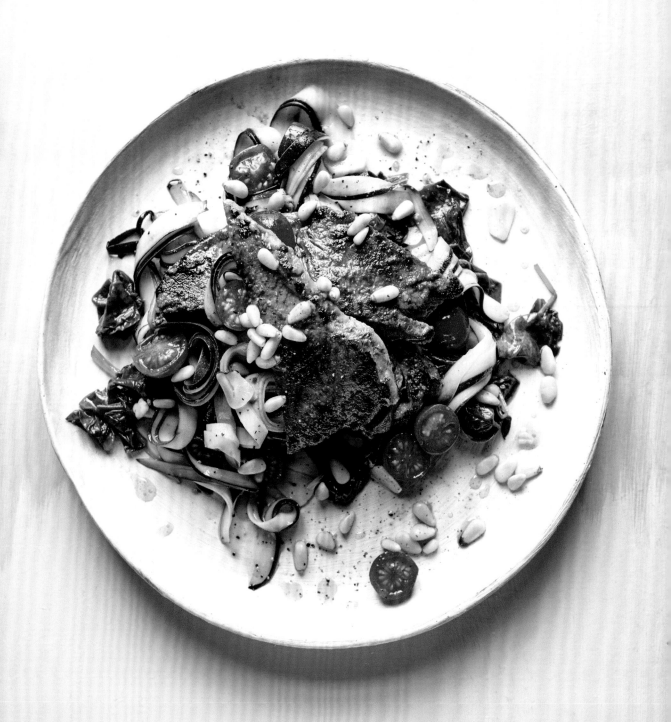

THAI SALMON AND COCONUT CURRY

REDUCED-CARB
MAKE AHEAD
GOOD TO FREEZE

INGREDIENTS

½ tbsp coconut oil
2 star anise
handful of coriander, leaves
  and stalks separated
1 lemongrass stalk, tender
  white part only, finely sliced
3 spring onions, finely sliced
1 red chilli, de-seeded and
  finely sliced
¼ aubergine, chopped into
  2cm chunks
50g green beans, roughly
  halved
2 tbsp Thai green curry paste
175ml coconut milk
1 x 150g skinless salmon fillet,
  chopped into 3cm chunks
4 raw king prawns, peeled and
  deveined
1 tbsp fish sauce
juice of 1 lime

Just when you didn't think I had another curry up my sleeve . . .
Remember, this is a low-carb recipe, so don't go adding rice
or noodles – just make sure you have loads of your favourite
veg instead.

METHOD

Melt the coconut oil in a large frying pan or wok over a medium
to high heat and add the star anise. Roughly chop up the
coriander stalks and fry with the star anise for about 30 seconds.

Add the lemongrass, spring onions, chilli, aubergine and
green beans and continue stir-frying for a further 3 minutes.

Spoon in the curry paste, mixing it in with the other ingredients,
and continue frying and stirring almost constantly for 1 minute.

Pour in the coconut milk and bring up to the boil. Simmer for
5 minutes and then gently plop the salmon pieces and prawns
into the pan. Continue simmering for a further 3–4 minutes,
or until you are happy the salmon is cooked through – you
can check this by slicing into one of the larger pieces to make
sure the flesh has turned matt pink in colour – but try not to
overcook it.

Take the pan off the heat and stir through the fish sauce,
lime juice and the coriander leaves. Serve up in a big bowl.

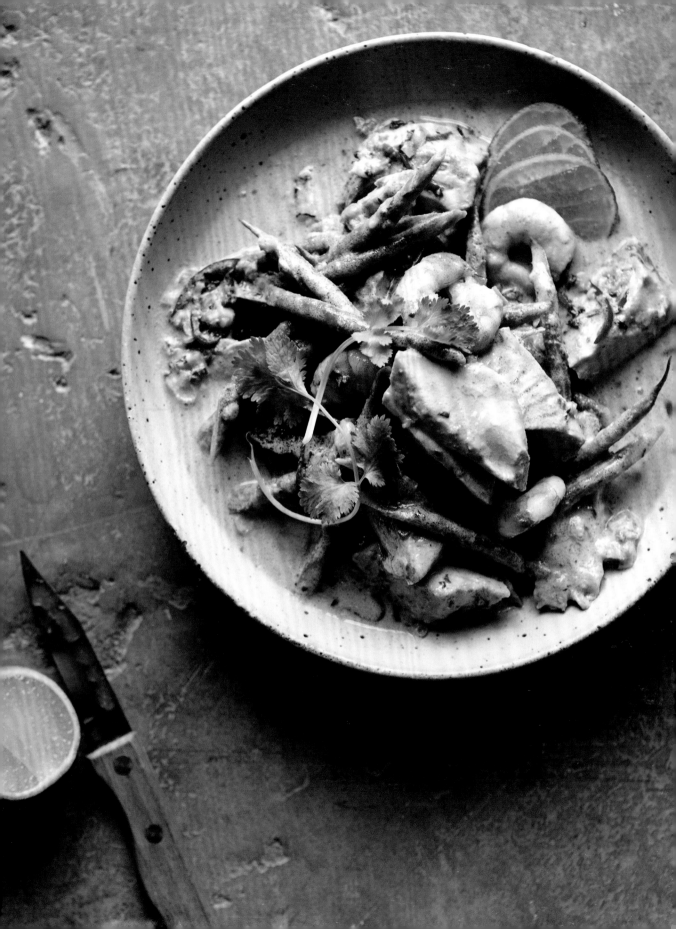

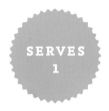

SALMON WITH WATERCRESS AND CASHEW PESTO

REDUCED-CARB
MAKE AHEAD
INGREDIENTS

1 lemon, halved
2 x 120g skinless salmon fillets
2 large handfuls of watercress,
   plus a little extra to serve
handful of basil
30 cashew nuts, roughly
   chopped
20ml olive oil
15g parmesan, grated
3 cherry tomatoes, halved,
   to serve

Pesto doesn't have to be just about basil and pine nuts.
I like to experiment and this one with cashews tastes wicked
on the salmon.

METHOD

Put a half-filled saucepan of water on to boil and squeeze in one
half of the lemon.

When the water is boiling, slide in the salmon fillets, put a lid on
the pan and reduce the heat to minimum. Cook the fish like this
for 3 minutes, then turn off the heat and leave in the warm water
until you're ready to eat.

While the fish is poaching, squeeze the juice of the second lemon
half into a blender and add the watercress, basil, cashew nuts,
olive oil and parmesan. Blitz until smooth. Depending on how
much watercress you have put in, you may need to add a little
warm water to get things moving.

When you are happy the salmon is cooked through, remove the
fillets from the saucepan and dab them dry on a piece of kitchen
roll. You can check the salmon is cooked by slicing into the thick
end of a fillet to make sure the flesh has turned matt pink in
colour.

Flake the fish onto a plate, drizzle over the pesto, top with the
extra watercress and serve with the cherry tomatoes.

LAMB CHOPS WITH HARISSA GUACAMOLE

SERVES 1

REDUCED-CARB INGREDIENTS

3 lamb chops
salt and pepper
1 ripe avocado, de-stoned
¼ red onion, diced
1 tbsp harissa – use more if
   you like it hot!
handful of coriander, roughly
   chopped
salt and pepper
¼ cucumber, de-seeded and
   chopped into chunks
25g toasted pine nuts
small green salad, to serve

If you haven't tried harissa before, you should defo give this dish a go. Trust me, the harissa kick in this guacamole goes brilliantly with the lamb and it is completely addictive!

METHOD

Preheat your grill to maximum.

Season the lamb with salt and pepper and place on a baking tray. Slide under the hot grill and cook the chops for about 7 minutes on each side before turning off the heat and leaving the lamb to rest.

While the chops are cooking, scoop the flesh of the avocado into a bowl and add the onion, harissa and coriander as well as a decent pinch of salt and pepper. Using the back of a fork, smash the ingredients together until they are well combined.

Plate up the chops next to a pile of the spicy guacamole, the cooling cucumber chunks and a good scattering of toasted pine nuts. Serve with a crisp green salad.

SERVES 1

CHICKEN SALAD WITH LEMON PESTO

A quick and easy salad that's great eaten cold so is perfect for taking to work – much better than buying a sandwich on the go and it will keep you lean, too.

REDUCED-CARB
MAKE AHEAD
INGREDIENTS

1 x 240g skinless chicken
   breast fillet
drizzle of olive oil
salt and pepper
1 tsp cumin seeds
25g pine nuts
1 tbsp pesto
juice of 1 lemon
large handful of baby spinach
   leaves, rocket or watercress
1 pre-cooked beetroot
5 sundried tomatoes, roughly
   halved
40g feta

METHOD

Preheat a griddle pan over a high heat.

Place the chicken between two pieces of cling film or baking parchment on a chopping board. Using a rolling pin, meat mallet or any other blunt instrument, bash the chicken until it is about 1cm thick all over.

Drizzle the breast with olive oil and season with salt and pepper. When the griddle pan is smoking hot, fry the bashed breast for about 4 minutes on each side. When you are happy the chicken is cooked through – you can check by slicing into a thicker part to make sure the meat is white all the way through, with no raw pink bits left – remove it to a plate and leave to rest.

While the chicken is cooking, toast the cumin seeds and pine nuts in a frying pan for about 1 minute over a high heat. Slide them onto a plate and leave to cool.

Dollop the pesto into a bowl, squeeze in the lemon juice and stir until thoroughly combined.

When you're ready to eat, lay the chicken on a plate and artistically chuck on the salad leaves, followed by the beetroot and sundried tomatoes. Crumble over the feta and drizzle the lemon pesto on top. Finish by scattering over the toasted seeds and nuts.

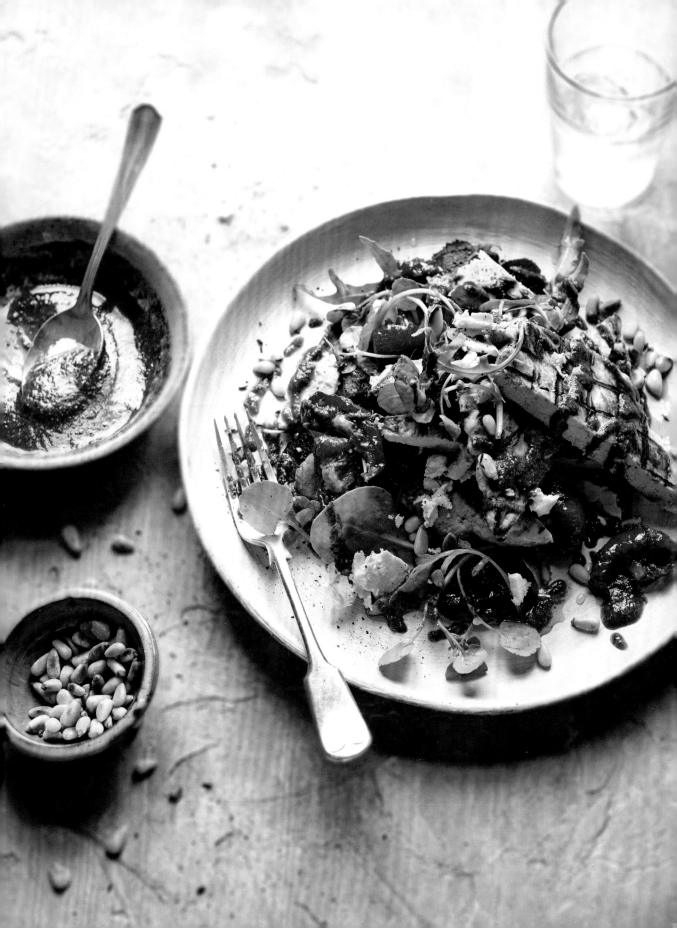

PORK TENDERLOIN WITH PEAR AND BLUE CHEESE

SERVES 1

With classic flavour combinations, this dish is packed full of the fats your body needs when resting. I like using pork tenderloin because when it's cooked in butter it doesn't dry out.

REDUCED-CARB INGREDIENTS

250g pork tenderloin, trimmed of visible fat
salt and pepper
1 tsp butter
2 sage leaves, finely sliced
1 pear, quartered and cored
large handful of rocket
large handful of baby spinach leaves
2 tsp olive oil
2 tsp red wine vinegar
40g gorgonzola, crumbed
15g walnuts, roughly chopped

METHOD

Place the pork between two pieces of cling film or baking parchment on a chopping board. Using a rolling pin, meat mallet or any other blunt instrument, bash the meat until it is about 1cm thick all over. Season the pork well with salt and pepper.

Melt the butter in a large frying pan over a medium to high heat. When bubbling, add the sage and leave for ten seconds before carefully laying the bashed pork in the pan and frying for 2–3 minutes on each side. To check that the pork is cooked, slice into a thick part of the meat to make sure there is no pink left.

While the pork is cooking, cut the pear quarters in half again to give yourself 8 pieces. Chuck the pear into a bowl and then add all the remaining ingredients. Using gentle hands, toss the salad together.

I like to lay my cooked pork down first and then pile the salad on top of it.

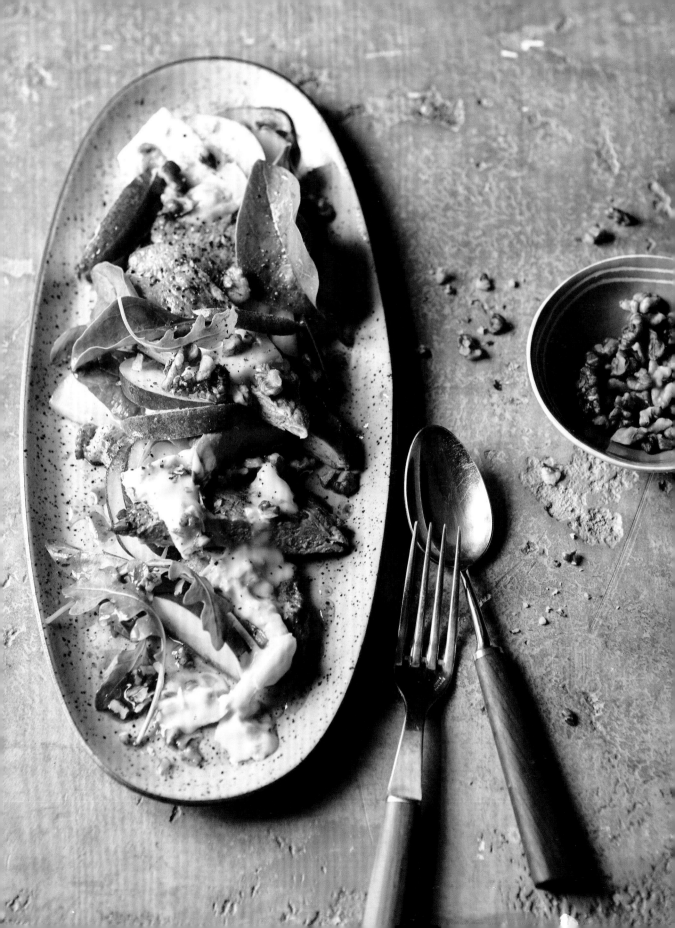

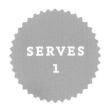

CHEESY HAM STUFFED CHICKEN

Gooey melted cheese and ham all wrapped up in a chicken breast? Errrm, yes please – sold! This is one of those 'tastes too good to be true' recipes that you will want to eat more than once a week.

REDUCED-CARB INGREDIENTS

1 x 220g skinless chicken breast fillet
salt and pepper
1 slice of deli-style ham
1 slice of cheddar (about 15g)
1 tsp butter
50ml chicken stock
4 midget trees (tender-stem broccoli), any bigger stalks sliced in half lengthways
50g green beans or mange tout
25ml double cream

METHOD

Put a saucepan of water on to boil.

Place the chicken between two pieces of cling film or baking parchment on a chopping board. Using a rolling pin, meat mallet or any other blunt instrument, bash the chicken until it is about 1cm thick all over.

Remove the top layer of cling film and season the chicken with salt and pepper. Imagine a line down the middle of the bashed fillet and lay the ham and then the slice of cheese just to the right of centre, ensuring there is a border all the way around. Now fold the left-hand side of the chicken over the ham and cheese and press against the right-hand side.

Melt the butter in a large frying pan over a medium to high heat and, when bubbling, gently lay in the chicken breast and leave it to brown on the bottom for about 4 minutes. Flip the fillet and pour in the chicken stock. Cover the pan with a lid (if you don't have one big enough then just use a plate, or a tray) and let the chicken cook away like this for about 4 more minutes.

Meanwhile, drop the midget trees and green beans or mange tout into the pan of boiling water and cook them for about 2½ minutes before draining in a colander.

Remove the lid from the frying pan and pour in the double cream. The cheese may well be oozing out of the fillet a little, but don't worry, the sauce will catch it. The chicken should be cooked through by now, but you can check this by slicing into the thick end to make sure the meat is white all the way through, with no raw pink bits left.

Serve up your stuffed chicken breast topped with the sauce and a side helping of the greens.

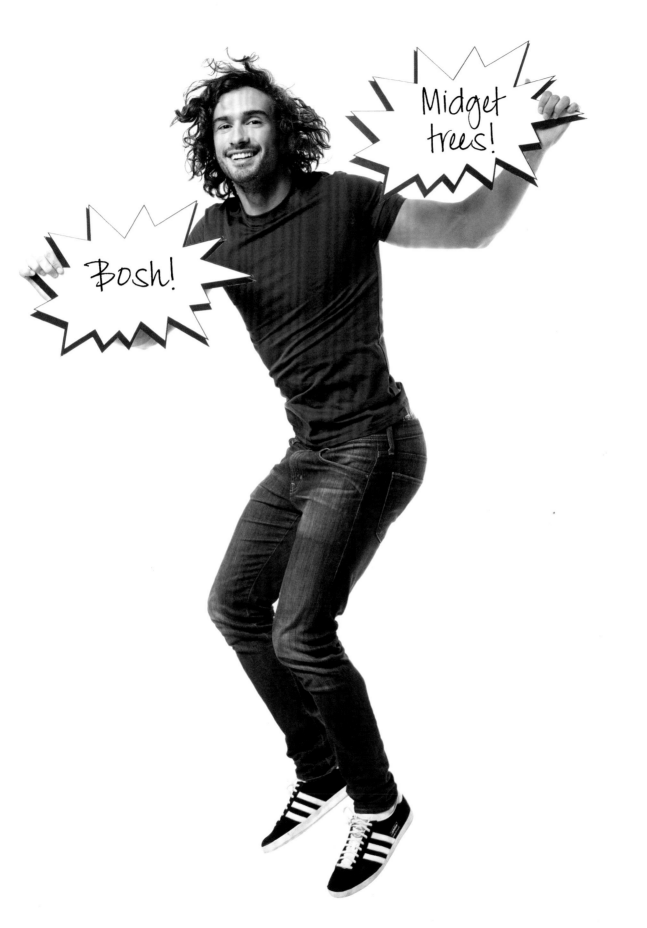

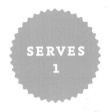

REDUCED-CARB
MAKE AHEAD
GOOD TO FREEZE

INGREDIENTS

1 tbsp coconut oil
1 cinnamon stick
½ red onion, sliced
½ aubergine, chopped into
  2cm chunks
4 midget trees (tender-stem
  broccoli), any bigger stalks
  sliced in half lengthways
1 red chilli, finely sliced
2 tbsp massaman curry paste
200ml coconut milk
1 x 240g skinless chicken
  breast fillet, sliced into 1cm
  strips
handful of coriander, roughly
  chopped
1 tbsp fish sauce
2 tbsp tamarind paste
2 tbsp desiccated coconut
lime wedges, to serve

MASSAMAN CURRY

Yeah, yeah, I know, a massaman is traditionally slow-cooked using beef and potatoes, but this is Lean in 15 and a reduced-carb meal, so I had to speed things up and cut out the potatoes. Don't worry, though – this curry with chicken tastes just as good, if not better.

METHOD

Melt half of the coconut oil in a large frying pan over a medium to high heat. Add the cinnamon, onion and aubergine and stir-fry for 2 minutes. Chuck in the midget trees and chilli and continue to stir-fry for another minute.

Dollop in the massaman paste and mix it through the other ingredients. Stir-fry for a further minute, stirring almost constantly, then pour in the coconut milk and simmer for 2 minutes.

While the coconut milk is simmering away, melt the remaining coconut oil in a second frying pan over a high heat. Fry the chicken for 2 minutes, browning it a little all over. Tip the chicken into the coconut curry mixture, bring it back up to the boil and simmer for 4 minutes, or until you are certain the chicken is fully cooked. Check by slicing into one of the larger pieces to make sure the meat is white all the way through, with no raw pink bits left.

Turn off the heat from under the pan and stir through the coriander, fish sauce, tamarind paste and desiccated coconut.

Serve up the mock massaman with wedges of lime.

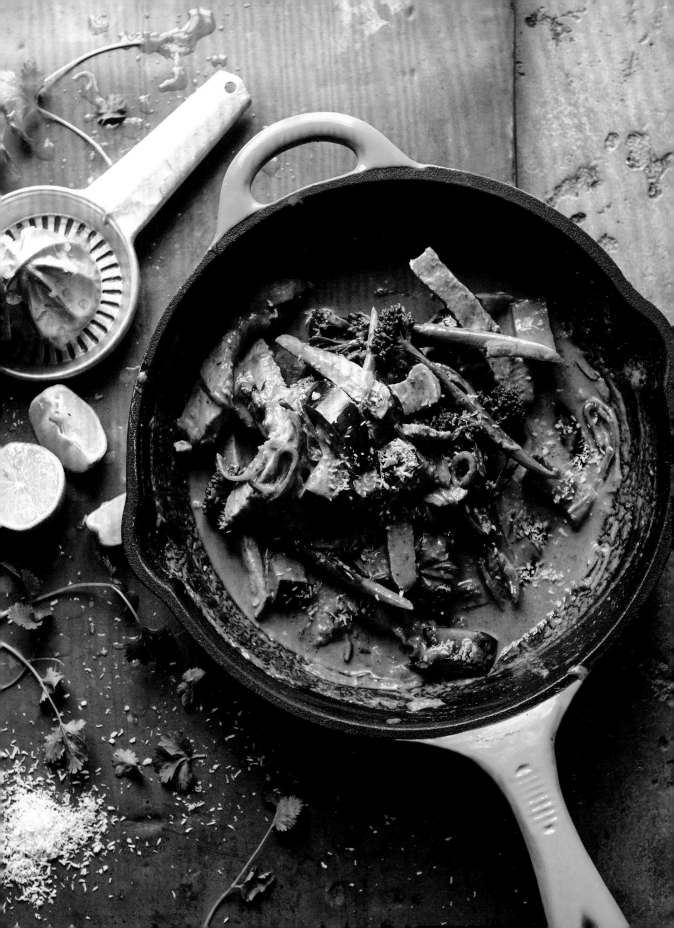

**SERVES
2**

REDUCED-CARB
MAKE AHEAD
LONGER RECIPE

INGREDIENTS

50ml reduced-fat Greek
  yoghurt
2 tbsp harissa
juice of 1 lemon
2 x 240g skinless chicken
  breast fillets
1 tbsp olive oil
2 sprigs of thyme
1 red onion, sliced into wedges
1 courgette, sliced into half-
  moons
salt and pepper
8 cherry tomatoes, on the vine
  if possible
1 ripe avocado, sliced
2 large handfuls of rocket
40g pine nuts – optional

HARISSA-BAKED CHICKEN WITH AVOCADO SALAD

If you're new to harissa, be careful – you might just become addicted to it. This dish will take 40 minutes, so give it a go at the weekend and enjoy.

METHOD

Preheat your oven to 190°C (fan 170°C, gas mark 5).

Mix together the yoghurt, harissa and half of the lemon juice. Smear all over the chicken and leave to one side.

Toss together the olive oil, thyme, onion and courgette with a good pinch of salt and pepper. Spread the vegetables over the base of a roasting tray.

Lay the spiced chicken on top of the vegetables and slide into the oven. Roast for 15 minutes, then place the tomatoes on the tray as well and continue to roast for a further 8 minutes, or until you are happy the chicken is fully cooked. Check by slicing into a thicker part to make sure the meat is white all the way through, with no raw pink bits left.

Serve up the roasted vegetables and chicken with a salad of avocado and rocket dressed with the remaining lemon juice, and finish with a scattering of pine nuts, if using.

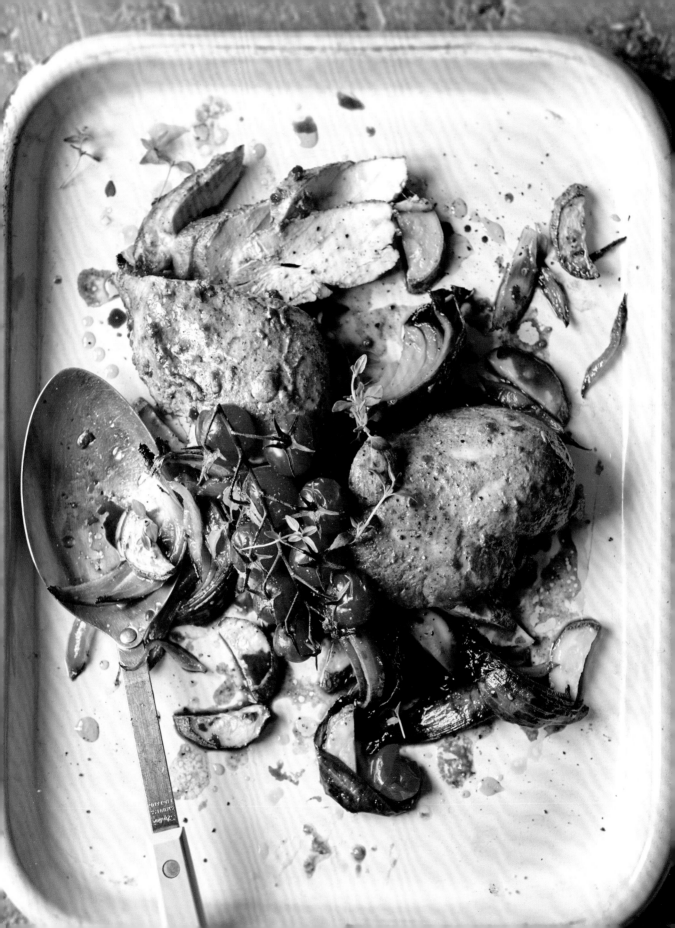

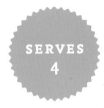

REDUCED-CARB
LONGER RECIPE

INGREDIENTS

2 tbsp coconut oil

1.25kg rump steak, chopped
 into large chunks

1 tsp butter

1 onion, diced

2 celery sticks, diced

1 carrot, diced

12 mushrooms, roughly
 chopped

2 sprigs of thyme

1 bay leaf

1½ tbsp tomato puree

3 tbsp Worcestershire sauce

500ml beef stock

1 tbsp cornflour

large handful of parsley,
 roughly chopped

4 sheets of filo pastry

drizzle of olive oil

steamed greens, to serve

JOE'S BEEF AND MUSHROOM PIE

Who remembers my chicken pie from Book 1? It was such a hit with people that I decided to make another one, but this time with beef and filo pastry. It takes longer than 15 minutes (more like 50) but the whole family will love this pie, so it's well worth the wait.

METHOD

Preheat your oven to 190°C (fan 170°C, gas mark 5).

Melt half of the coconut oil in a large pan or casserole dish over a high heat. Add half of the meat to the pan, brown it all over and remove to a plate. Repeat the process with the remaining coconut oil and meat.

Dollop the butter into the same pan and melt it over a medium to high heat. When bubbling, add the onion, celery, carrot and mushrooms and fry, stirring occasionally, for about 5 minutes. Drop in the thyme and bay leaf and continue to fry for another minute.

Return the cooked meat to the pan and squeeze in the tomato puree. Stir-fry for 1 minute and then pour in the Worcestershire sauce and stock. Bring to a gentle simmer.

Mix the cornflour with 1 tablespoon of water and then stir it into the beef mixture. It should thicken pretty quickly. Tip the whole lot into a baking dish and leave to cool for 10 minutes.

Take the filo pastry out of the fridge, crumple the individual sheets into loose balls and place straight on top of the cooling stew so that it is entirely covered.

Drizzle the pastry with olive oil and then bake in the oven for 20 minutes, or until the pastry is browned and crisp.

Serve up with mounds of steamed green veg.

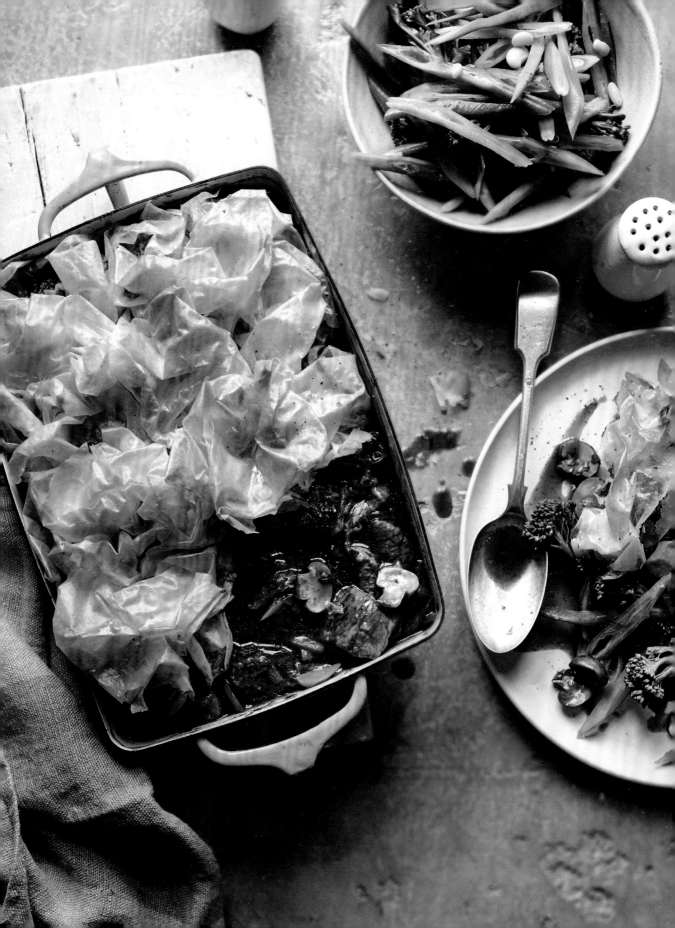

CHICKEN IN A BAG

A properly easy meal for the whole family to enjoy together. I'm using chicken thighs here because they have more flavour than breast fillets and we have the luxury of more time on this recipe (it will take an hour). They are also a lot cheaper. Feel free to add your favourite root vegetables to the mix.

REDUCED-CARB
LONGER RECIPE
INGREDIENTS

1 carrot, thinly sliced on the
   diagonal
1 parsnip, thinly sliced on the
   diagonal
1 courgette, thinly sliced on
   the diagonal
2 red onions, finely sliced
3 cloves garlic, crushed
3 sprigs of thyme
5 sage leaves, finely sliced
3 tomatoes, roughly chopped
80g chorizo, chopped into
   1cm cubes
salt and pepper
1 tsp butter
12 skinless and boneless
   chicken thighs
125ml chicken stock
large handful of parsley,
   roughly chopped
juice of 2 lemons
50g parmesan, grated
50g pine nuts – optional
a few handfuls of baby
   spinach leaves, to serve

METHOD

Preheat your oven to 180°C (fan 160°C, gas mark 4).

Roll out a really big piece of foil, about 60cm in length, then rip out a similar-sized piece of baking parchment. Lay the foil on a flat baking tray, then place the parchment on top of the foil.

Toss the carrot, parsnip, courgette, onions, garlic, thyme, sage, tomatoes and chorizo together in a bowl, adding a good pinch of salt and pepper.

Rub the butter onto the baking parchment, greasing a rectangle about 40 x 20cm in the middle. Pile the vegetable mixture onto the buttered rectangle, then arrange the chicken thighs on top of the veg.

Cut a second piece of foil the same size as the first and place over everything. Crimp the edges of the foil together to seal the parcel, leaving one small gap. Carefully pour the stock into that gap, seal it up, then slide the tray into the oven and bake for 40 minutes.

Remove the tray from the oven and let everything sit for 5 minutes. Then, to be dramatic, cut open the foil at the table and sprinkle the contents with the chopped parsley, several good squeezes of lemon juice, the parmesan and the pine nuts, if using. Pile baby spinach onto the serving plates and spoon the chicken and veg on top.

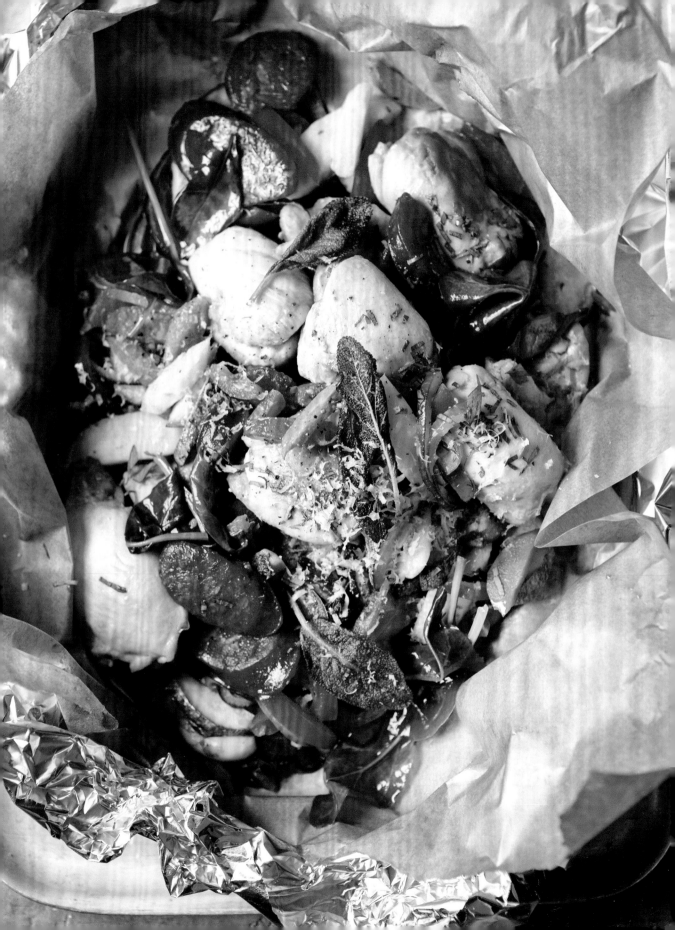

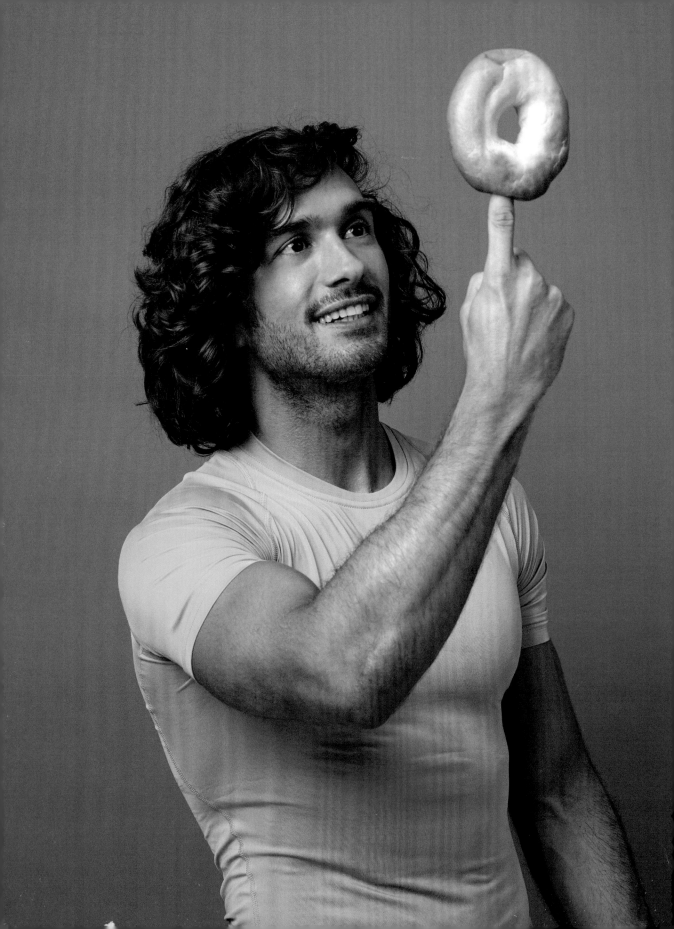

POST-WORKOUT RECIPES

4

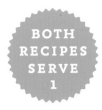

BANANA AND CHOCOLATE OVERNIGHT OATS

POST-WORKOUT
MAKE AHEAD
LONGER RECIPE
(quick to make but needs
8 hours' soaking time)

INGREDIENTS

250ml almond milk
2 scoops (60g) vanilla protein
  powder
1 ripe banana, roughly
  chopped
½ tbsp cocoa powder (over
  70% cocoa)
75g rolled oats
a little grated dark chocolate,
  to serve

Just like cheese and wine, chocolate and banana were made for each other. This is a great way to use up bananas that are going black. As they overripen, they become softer and sweeter, both great things for the overall taste of this brekkie.

METHOD

Place all the ingredients apart from the rolled oats and dark chocolate in a blender and blitz until smooth.

Pour the mixture over the oats and stir well. Leave to soak in a sealable container in the fridge for at least 8 hours, or overnight.

When you're ready to eat, sprinkle the dark chocolate over the top.

QUINOA OVERNIGHT OATS

POST-WORKOUT
MAKE AHEAD
LONGER RECIPE
(quick to make but needs
8 hours' soaking time)

INGREDIENTS

40g rolled oats
125g cooked quinoa
2 scoops (60g) vanilla protein
  powder
250ml almond milk
½ tsp ground cinnamon
3 dried apricots, roughly
  chopped
2 tbsp raisins
1 tbsp honey

This one's going to keep you full up until lunch, that's for sure. The combination of cooked quinoa and oats gives it a really nice nutty flavour.

METHOD

Tip all the ingredients apart from the apricots, raisins and honey into a large bowl and mix well. Pour the mix into a sealable container and leave to soak in the fridge for at least 8 hours, or overnight.

When you're ready to eat, remove the lid and top with the dried apricots, raisins and a drizzle of honey.

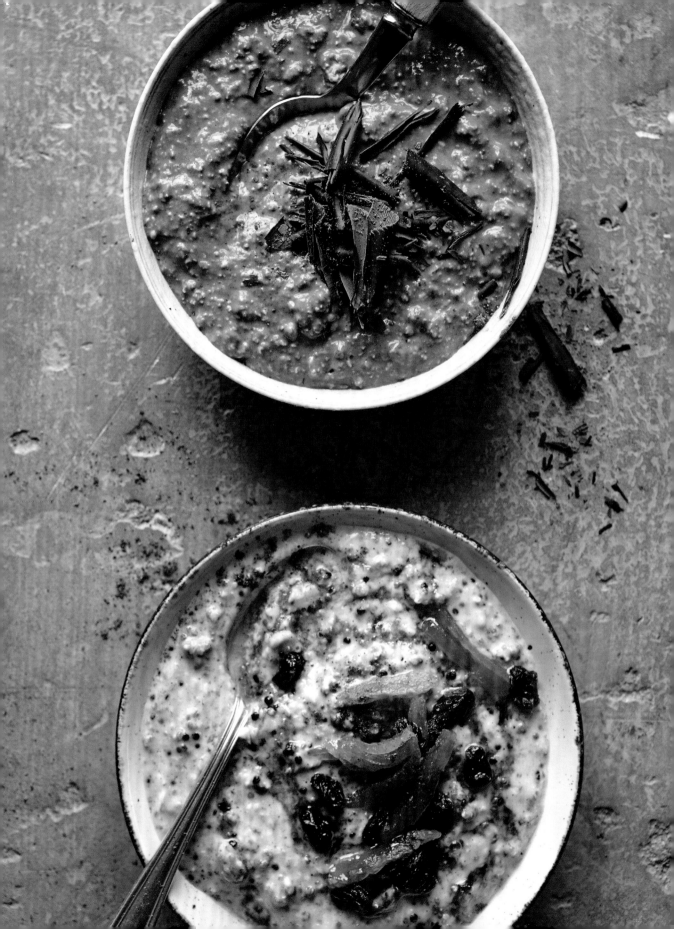

PEACH MELBA SMOOTHIE

This is one of my favourite smoothie recipes in the book. Great to have after an early morning workout and ready in minutes.

METHOD

Place all the ingredients in a blender and blitz until smooth.

SERVES 1

POST-WORKOUT

INGREDIENTS

1 peach, roughly chopped
1 banana, roughly chopped
small handful of raspberries
2 scoops (60g) vanilla protein powder
50g porridge oats
200ml water
small handful of ice

PORRIDGE AND MALT SMOOTHIE

Here's one for those days when you've smashed a workout but don't fancy cooking. It is quick and gives you all the macronutrients your body needs to refuel.

METHOD

Place all the ingredients in a blender and blitz until smooth.

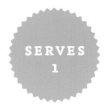

SERVES 1

POST-WORKOUT

INGREDIENTS

75g porridge oats
2 scoops (60g) vanilla or chocolate protein powder
100ml almond milk
75ml water
1½ tbsp malt powder (I use Horlicks)

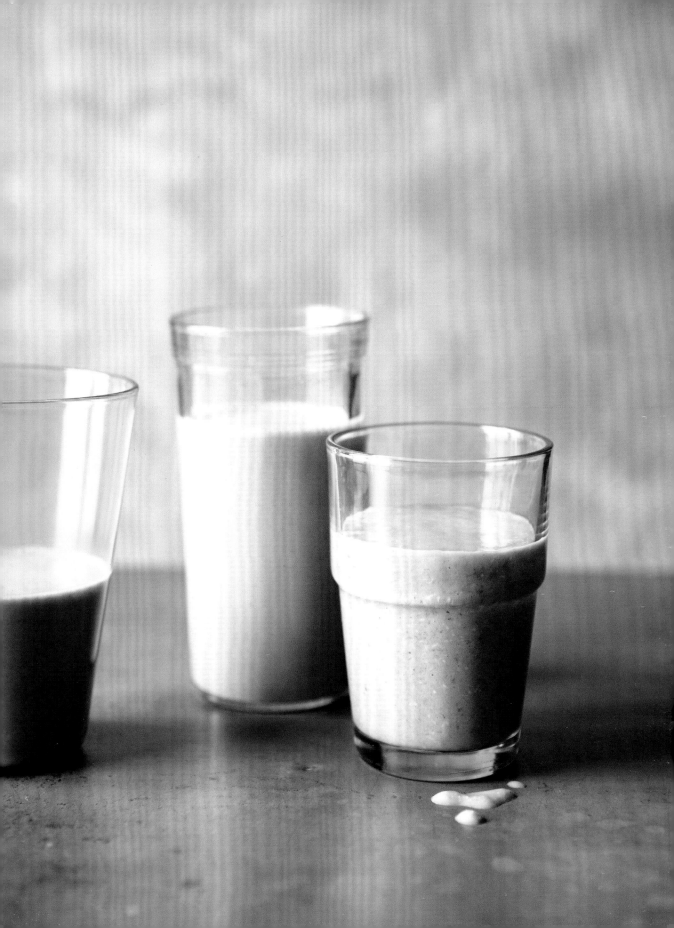

COCOBERRY OATS

POST-WORKOUT
INGREDIENTS

125g rolled oats
600ml coconut water
2 scoops (60g) vanilla protein
  powder
small handful each of
  blueberries and raspberries,
  to serve
drizzle of honey, to serve

You might think I'm mad using coconut water in my porridge, but you'll understand why when you try it. If you train early in the morning and need a quick and easy refuel meal, then this is perfect for you.

METHOD

Tip the oats into a saucepan, pour in the coconut water and bring to a simmer over a medium heat. Make sure you stir regularly to stop the oats from sticking to the base of the pan and burning.

Cook the oats for about 10 minutes, or until they are totally tender and the porridge has become thick and creamy.

Remove the pan from the heat and stir through the protein powder.

Serve up the porridge topped with fresh berries and a drizzle of honey.

POST-WORKOUT
GOOD TO FREEZE
INGREDIENTS

125g buckwheat flour
1 banana, roughly chopped
½ tsp ground cinnamon
2 scoops (60g) vanilla protein
  powder
1 egg
175ml almond milk
1 tbsp coconut oil
dollop of reduced-fat Greek
  yoghurt, to serve
small handful each of
  raspberries and blueberries,
  to serve
drizzle of honey, to serve

GET STACKED PROTEIN PANCAKES

There's nothing more rewarding after a workout than a giant stack of protein pancakes. I visualize these when I'm training to keep me motivated. It works every time! And with buckwheat they are super-healthy. #PancakeMe.

METHOD

Place the buckwheat flour, banana, cinnamon, protein powder, egg and almond milk into a food processor and blitz until smooth.

Melt a little of the coconut oil in a large non-stick frying pan over a medium to high heat. Pour in small puddles of the pancake mixture (about 1½ tablespoons each). The mixture should spread and form a little circle on its own. I normally manage three pancakes comfortably in my pan, or four if I'm in a rush.

Cook the pancakes for about 2 minutes, by which time bubbles should rise to the surface and pop – this is the sign to flip the pancakes. Carefully flip them and cook for a further 2 minutes on the other side.

Remove the cooked pancakes to a clean sheet of kitchen roll to remove any excess oil. Repeat the process with the remaining pancakes, then stack them high, dollop on the yoghurt, scatter over the berries and finish with a drizzle of honey.

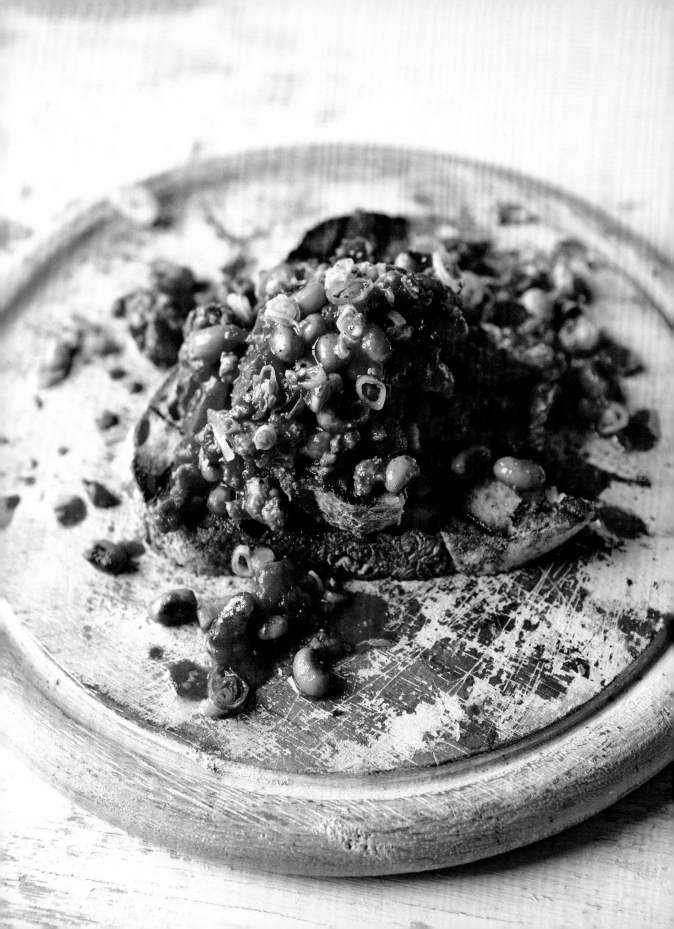

SPICED TURKEY AND BEANS ON TOAST

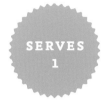

POST-WORKOUT
INGREDIENTS

½ tbsp coconut oil
2 spring onions, sliced
200g turkey mince
2 tsp smoked paprika
1 tbsp sherry or balsamic
   vinegar
175g tinned chopped tomatoes
200g tinned black-eyed beans,
   drained and rinsed
1 thick slice of crusty bread,
   toasted

If you train early in the morning, this is an awesome post-workout breakfast. But everyone knows bread makes you fat, right? LOL. I'm joking – of course it doesn't. So go get yourself a nice big chunky slice of your favourite bread and enjoy it.

METHOD

Melt the coconut oil in a large frying pan over a high heat. Add the spring onions and fry for 30 seconds, then tip in the turkey.

Fry the turkey, breaking up large lumps with a wooden spoon, for about 2–3 minutes until most of the meat has turned from raw pink to cooked white. Sprinkle in the paprika and continue cooking and stirring for a further minute, then pour in the vinegar which will bubble up and evaporate to almost nothing.

Tip the tomatoes and beans into the pan, bring the whole lot to the boil and simmer for about 10 minutes, or until you are sure the turkey is totally cooked through.

Serve up your turkey and beans on a thick piece of toasted bread.

SERVES 1

INGREDIENTS

1 large potato
½ tbsp coconut oil
2 spring onions, finely sliced
1 red chilli, de-seeded and
  finely sliced
3 cherry tomatoes, halved
1 x 180g skinless chicken
  breast fillet, sliced into 1cm
  strips
2 eggs
2 tsp rose harissa
2 large handfuls of spinach
black pepper

CHICKEN WITH HASH BROWNS

If you've ever eaten breakfast in an American diner, you'll know they often have their own version of sautéed potatoes. This is the Body Coach version and I'm sure you'll be coming back for more.

METHOD

Put a saucepan of water on to boil.

Grate the potato, skin and all. Give the grated flesh a good squeeze over the sink to remove some of the liquid.

Melt half of the coconut oil in a small non-stick frying pan over a medium to high heat and drop in the grated potato. Use the back of a spatula to flatten it out across the base of the pan. Fry the potato for about 5 minutes on each side, reducing the heat a little if you think the potato is burning.

Meanwhile, melt the remaining coconut oil in a second frying pan and chuck in the spring onions, chilli, tomatoes and chicken and stir-fry for 4–5 minutes, or until you are happy the chicken is fully cooked. Check by slicing into one of the larger pieces to make sure the meat is white all the way through, with no raw pink bits left.

Carefully crack the eggs into the hot water to poach, reducing the heat until the water is just 'burping'. Cook the eggs for about 4 minutes for a runny yolk, then lift out carefully with a slotted spoon and drain on kitchen roll.

When you are happy the meat is cooked through, add the harissa and spinach to the frying pan and toss together with the other ingredients until fully wilted.

Slide the hash brown onto a piece of kitchen roll and dab it to remove any excess oil, then plate it up. Top with the chicken and spinach mix and finish with the poached eggs and a pinch of black pepper.

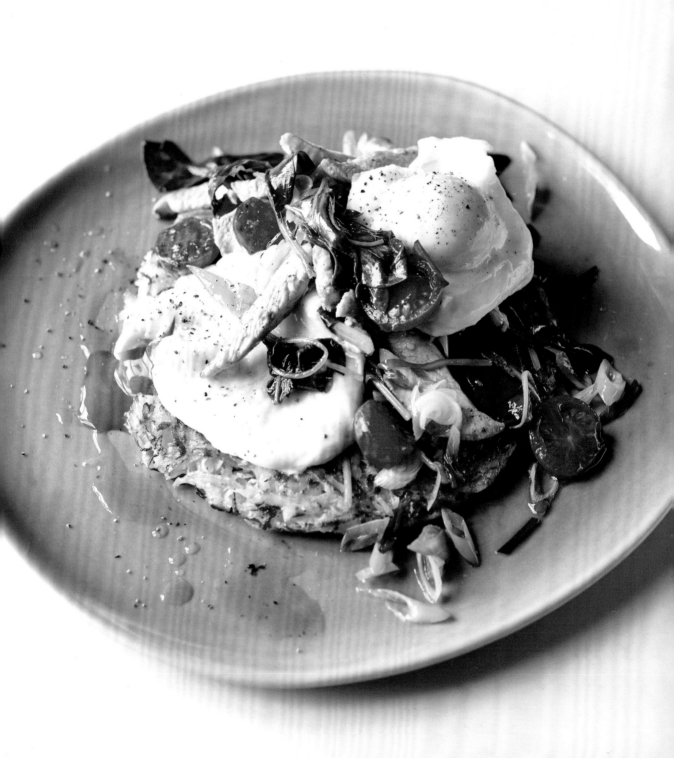

SMOKY BEANS ON TOAST WITH CHICKEN SAUSAGES

SERVES 1

POST-WORKOUT
INGREDIENTS

4 chicken sausages
1 tbsp butter
¼ red onion, diced
3 chestnut mushrooms,
  roughly chopped
200g tinned cannellini beans,
  drained and rinsed
1 tbsp tomato puree
1 tsp smoked paprika
large handful of baby spinach
  leaves
1 thick slice of toast

I used to live on beans on toast as a kid, so I thought I would make a healthy version. It may not be covered in tomato ketchup but it still tastes awesome. Chicken sausages are becoming much more popular nowadays, so you should be able to find them in your local supermarket.

METHOD

Preheat your grill to maximum. Lay the sausages on a baking tray and slide them under the hot grill. Cook them for about 12 minutes, turning them regularly, by which time they should be cooked through. Check by slicing into one to make sure the meat is white all the way through, with no raw pink bits left.

While the sausages are cooking, melt the butter in a frying pan over a medium to high heat. When bubbling, chuck in the onion and mushrooms and stir-fry for about 4 minutes, or until the onion has softened a little and the mushrooms have browned a bit.

Add the cannellini beans, tomato puree and smoked paprika to the pan, and toss the whole lot together. Cook for a further minute or so and then pour in 50ml of water. Bring to the boil, then reduce to a simmer and cook for 2 minutes. Drop in the baby spinach and stir it through until totally wilted.

Serve the beans on a thick piece of toast with the sausages alongside.

POST-WORKOUT
MAKE AHEAD
INGREDIENTS

½ tbsp coconut oil

2 spring onions, finely sliced

1 x 220g sirloin steak, trimmed
of visible fat and sliced into
1cm strips

1 jarred red pepper, drained
and roughly sliced

4 cherry tomatoes, roughly
halved

1 tsp dried oregano

large handful of baby spinach
leaves

handful of coriander, roughly
chopped

2 medium tortillas

small green salad, to serve

QUESADILLA

I love a quesadilla and this one with sirloin steak really hits
the spot. Unfortunately, it's not a cheesy one because it's
important to keep the fat content lower in post-workout
meals, but it still tastes banging.

METHOD

Melt the coconut oil in a large frying pan over a high heat.
Chuck in the spring onions and fry for 30 seconds, then add
the meat and fry, stirring regularly, for 3 minutes.

Add the red pepper and cherry tomatoes. Stir-fry for 2 minutes,
by which time the tomatoes should be starting to soften. Turn
down the heat to medium and sprinkle in the dried oregano,
baby spinach and coriander. Keep cooking until the spinach has
totally wilted.

Heat a second frying pan over a medium to high heat. When
hot, lay a tortilla in the dry pan and pile on the steak mixture,
topping with the second tortilla and pressing it down a little
with the back of a spatula. Dry-fry the quesadilla like this for
about 2 minutes.

Now comes the tricky part – flipping. I find the best way is to
position a large plate on top and put my hand on it, then in
one swift movement to turn the frying pan upside down so
the quesadilla drops onto the plate. Put the frying pan back
on the heat and then slide the flipped quesadilla into the pan –
hey presto.

Cook the quesadilla for 2–3 minutes on the second side,
then slide it onto a chopping board, wedge up with a knife
and serve with a small green side salad.

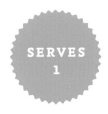

POST-WORKOUT
MAKE AHEAD
INGREDIENTS

½ tbsp coconut oil

½ red onion, sliced into 6 thin
  wedges

1 x 240g sirloin steak, trimmed
  of visible fat and sliced into
  1cm strips

5 cherry tomatoes, halved

1 tsp smoked paprika

1 tsp dried oregano

½ tsp cayenne pepper

50g tinned kidney beans,
  drained and rinsed

1 jarred red pepper, drained
  and thinly sliced

2 medium pitta breads

shredded iceberg lettuce,
  to serve

¼ cucumber, roughly chopped
  into 2cm chunks, to serve

lemon wedges, to serve

THE BIG McLEANIE PITTA

If you're not in the mood for a workout, just look at this recipe.
I mean, how can you not want to go and train right now if
you get to smash this afterwards? #GetGoing.

METHOD

Melt the coconut oil in a large frying pan over a medium to
high heat. Add the onion and stir-fry for 30 seconds.

Chuck in the steak and cherry tomatoes and fry, stirring
every now and then, for about 2 minutes, or until the steak is
starting to colour a little and the tomatoes begin to soften.

Reduce the heat to medium and sprinkle in the paprika,
oregano and cayenne pepper, quickly followed by the kidney
beans and red pepper. Stir-fry everything together for 1 minute,
or until you are happy the beans are warmed through and the
steak is cooked how you like it (I like mine just a little rare).

Toast your pitta breads, slice them open and cram with the
steak mix. Top with the shredded lettuce and chunky cucumber
pieces, and serve with lemon wedges to squeeze over.

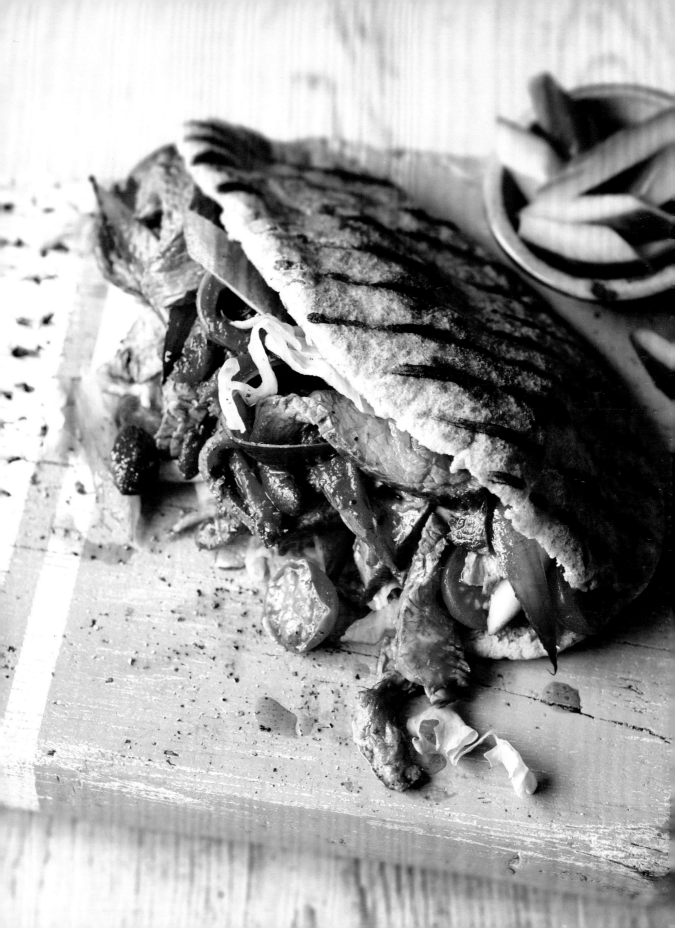

CHICKEN AND PINEAPPLE FRIED RICE

SERVES 1

POST-WORKOUT INGREDIENTS

2 tsp coconut oil

3 spring onions, finely sliced

2cm ginger, finely chopped

1 x 240g skinless chicken breast fillet, sliced into 1cm strips

50g spring greens, stalks removed and leaves shredded

250g pre-cooked brown rice

75g fresh or tinned pineapple chunks

1 tbsp light soy sauce

2 tsp sesame oil

handful of coriander, roughly chopped

small handful of beansprouts

As I always say, you've got to eat your greens and this dish contains plenty of them. It may seem like an odd combo but the sweetness of the pineapple is a great match with the nuttiness of the brown rice.

METHOD

Melt the coconut oil in a large frying pan or wok over a high heat. Chuck in the spring onions, ginger and chicken and stir-fry for about 2 minutes, by which time the chicken should be lightly browned and almost cooked.

Add the spring greens and toss together with the rest of the ingredients. Continue stir-frying for 1 minute then add the rice, crumbling it between your fingers as you drop it in, followed swiftly by 2 tablespoons of water, which will steam up to help warm through and separate the rice as well as finish the cooking of both the chicken and greens.

Keep stir-frying until you are happy the chicken is fully cooked and the rice is hot. Check the chicken is cooked by slicing into one of the larger pieces to make sure the meat is white all the way through, with no raw pink bits left.

Turn off the heat and add the pineapple chunks, soy sauce, sesame oil and coriander. Toss the whole lot together, then pile it high on a plate. Finish with a nice pile of crunchy beansprouts.

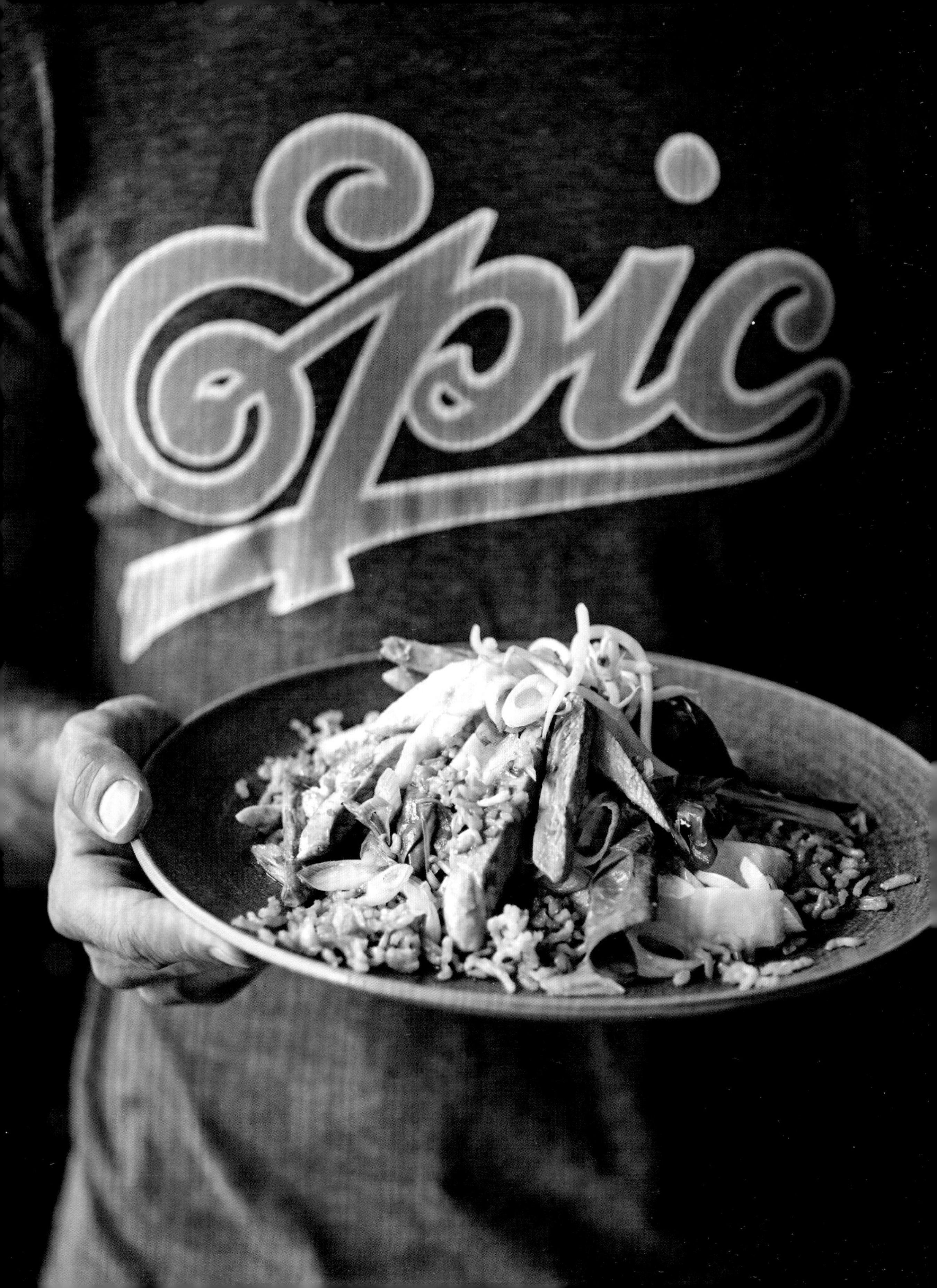
Epic

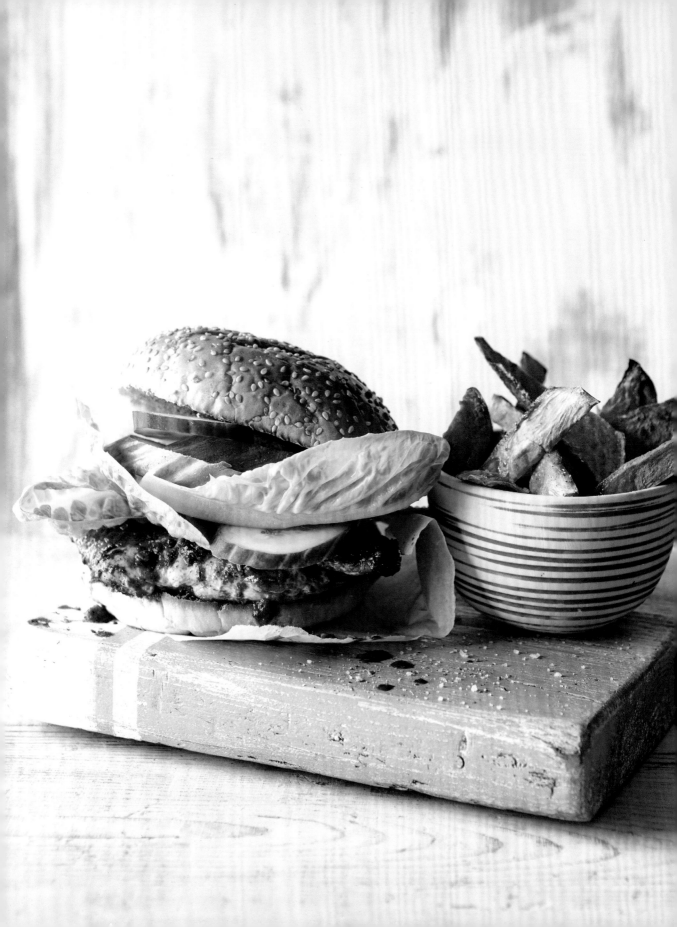

PIRI PIRI BUTTERFLY CHICKEN BURGER

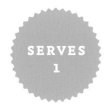

SERVES 1

POST-WORKOUT INGREDIENTS

1 sweet potato, peeled and sliced into 6 wedges

1 x 240g skinless chicken breast fillet

1 tbsp coconut oil

1 tbsp chipotle paste

juice of 1 lime

2 tsp Jamaican jerk seasoning

1 large burger bun

4 chunky slices of cucumber, to serve

2 big lettuce leaves, to serve

In case you didn't know, I'm a massive fan of burgers and piri piri chicken. So I thought why not combine the two and make this banging burger? This is a proper champion refuel meal, so smash your workout today and reward yourself.

METHOD

Zap the sweet potato wedges in your microwave for 4 minutes, rest for 2 minutes, then blast for another 4 minutes.

Meanwhile, place the chicken between two pieces of cling film or baking parchment on a chopping board. Using a rolling pin, meat mallet or any other blunt instrument, bash the chicken until it is about 1cm thick all over.

Melt half of the coconut oil in a frying pan over a medium to high heat. Carefully lay the bashed chicken in the pan and fry for about 4 minutes.

While the chicken is frying, mix together the chipotle, lime juice and jerk seasoning. When the chicken has had 4 minutes, flip it and pour half the chipotle mix over the breast, then cook for a further 4 minutes. Flip again, pour over the remaining chipotle mix and fry for a further 2 minutes on each side, by which time the chicken should be cooked through. Check by slicing into a thicker part to make sure the meat is white all the way through, with no raw pink bits left. Now remove the chicken to a plate to rest.

Melt the remaining coconut oil in a second frying pan over a medium to high heat and fry the sweet potatoes until they are golden brown all over.

Next, cut the bun in half and toast briefly in a toaster. Now you're ready to build your burger: lay the chicken breast on the bun base, top with cucumber and lettuce and then add the lid.

Serve up your burger and wedges – after that cooking workout you deserve every mouthful!

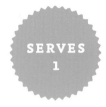

POST-WORKOUT
MAKE AHEAD
INGREDIENTS

1 medium potato, peeled
  and diced
60g frozen peas
2 x 125g sea bass fillets,
  skin on
salt
4 cherry tomatoes
50g plain flour
1 tsp turmeric
1 tsp curry powder
1 egg
½ tbsp coconut oil
handful of baby spinach leaves,
  to serve
lime wedges, to serve

SEA BASS WITH SPICED PEA AND POTATO CAKES

If potatoes are your favourite carb then these cakes will be right up your street. They've got a spicy little kick to them and taste unreal with the crispy sea bass.

METHOD

Put the kettle on to boil and preheat your grill to maximum.

Put the potato in a microwaveable bowl and pour over about 30ml of boiling water from the kettle. Cover with cling film and zap in the microwave for 3 minutes. Leave to rest for 1 minute and zap again for 3 minutes. Add the frozen peas and zap for another 3 minutes.

While the potato is in the microwave, lay the sea bass fillets, skin side up, on a baking tray. Season with a little salt and place the cherry tomatoes next to the fish.

Slide the tray under the grill and cook for about 7 minutes without turning. The tomatoes should be tender and cooked while still holding their shape, and the fish should be perfectly cooked under the crisp skin. Make sure the fish is done by checking that the flesh has turned from a raw pale colour to cooked bright white, then turn off the grill and leave the fillets to keep warm until you're ready to eat.

By now the potato and peas should have finished in the microwave. Drain off any excess water and roughly mash them together.

Beat in the plain flour, turmeric, curry powder and egg. Melt the coconut oil in a frying pan over a medium to high heat. Form two large patties with the potato mix and lay them carefully in the hot oil. Fry for about 2 minutes on each side until they are golden brown.

Plate up the spuds, carefully remove the sea bass skin and place the fillets on your plate along with the tomatoes, a handful of baby spinach leaves and some fresh lime wedges.

KOREAN CHICKEN RICE BOWL

POST-WORKOUT
MAKE AHEAD
INGREDIENTS

½ tbsp coconut oil
1 x 240g skinless chicken
   breast fillet, sliced into 1cm
   strips
2 cloves garlic, 1 finely sliced
2 spring onions, finely sliced
250g pre-cooked brown rice
large handful of baby spinach
   leaves
50g beansprouts
¼ tsp sesame oil
1½ tbsp light soy sauce
2 tsp rice vinegar
½ red chilli, de-seeded and
   sliced, to serve – optional

Never tried Korean food before? No worries, it's really simple to make and packed with flavours you probably love, like garlic, chilli and soy sauce. I've gone for brown rice in this recipe because I like the nuttiness, but you can use any rice you like.

METHOD

Put the kettle on to boil.

Melt the coconut oil in a frying pan over a high heat. Scrape in the chicken and stir-fry for 2 minutes, then add the sliced garlic and half of the spring onions. Continue to stir-fry for 2–3 minutes until you are happy the chicken is fully cooked. Check by slicing into one of the larger pieces to make sure the meat is white all the way through, with no raw pink bits left.

While the chicken is cooking, zap the rice in the microwave according to the packet instructions.

Drop the baby spinach and beansprouts into a colander and pour over the boiled water from the kettle to wilt the vegetables. Run a little cold water over them until they're cool enough to handle. Squeeze the wilted veg to remove as much excess water as possible and then chuck them into a bowl.

Pour the sesame oil over the veg, grate in the remaining garlic clove, and then add half of the soy sauce to the chicken and the other half in with the vegetables.

Tip the brown rice into a bowl, sprinkle over the rice vinegar and then top with the cooked chicken and the wilted veg salad. Finish with a fiery topping of red chilli, if using.

POST-WORKOUT
INGREDIENTS

350ml chicken stock
3cm ginger, roughly bashed
1 lemongrass stalk, white part
  only, bashed with the side
  of a knife
1 red chilli, slit open – remove
  the seeds if you don't like
  it hot
250g pre-cooked egg noodles
1 pak choi, quartered
  lengthways
40g mange tout
240g cooked skinless chicken
  breast, shredded or sliced
juice of 1 lime
1 tbsp fish sauce
40g beansprouts
handful each of coriander and
  mint, leaves only

CHICKEN PHO

Who knows how to pronounce 'pho'? Is it foo, fo or po? It's actually 'fuh', but don't worry about the name, just make this dish and dive in. It's a really good way of using up leftover cooked meats, so try it with chicken, beef or pork.

METHOD

Pour the stock into a saucepan and add the ginger, lemongrass and chilli and bring to the boil. Simmer for about 5 minutes to let the stock infuse with all the flavourings.

Put the kettle on to boil and tip the noodles into a colander over a sink. Pour the boiling water over the noodles – this helps not only to warm them through but also to remove some of the oil these noodles are sometimes packed in. Shake the noodles to drain off the excess water, then carefully place them in the base of a large bowl.

Add the pak choi and the mange tout to the stock and boil for 2 minutes.

While the vegetables are cooking, lay the cooked chicken on top of the warmed noodles.

Take the stock off the heat and stir through half of the lime juice and the fish sauce. It's not totally necessary, but you might want to remove the ginger, chilli and lemongrass from the stock before pouring the liquid and vegetables over the chicken and noodles.

Top the whole lot with the beansprouts, fresh herbs and remaining lime juice.

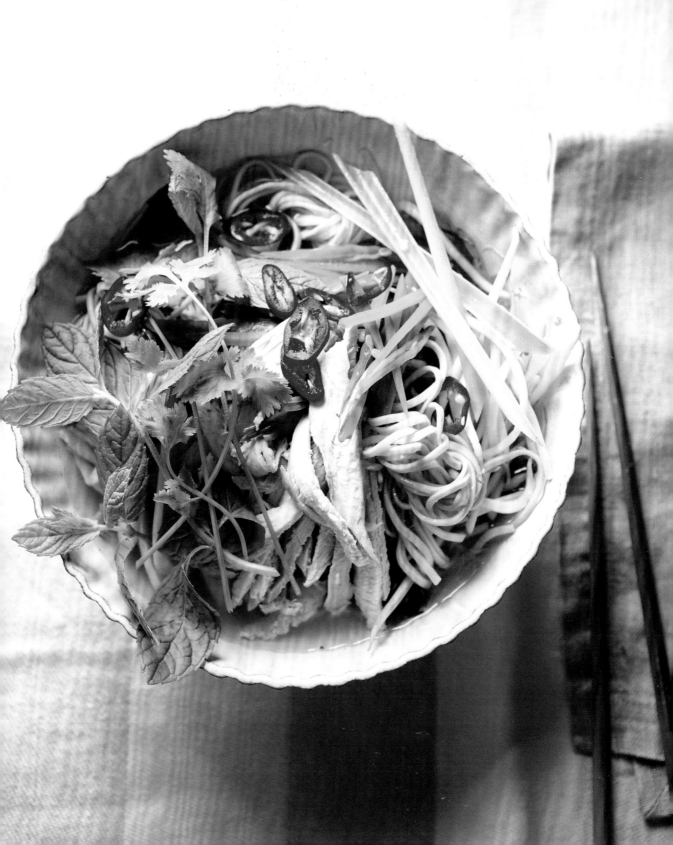

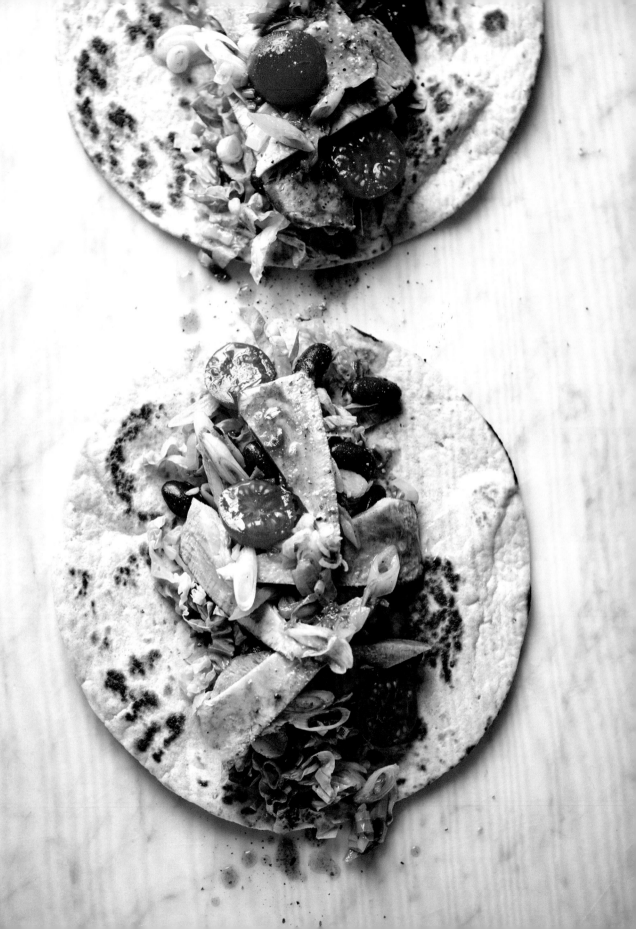

POST-WORKOUT
MAKE AHEAD
INGREDIENTS

½ tbsp coconut oil

3 spring onions, finely sliced

1 clove garlic, finely sliced

1 x 240g tuna steak, chopped
into 2–3cm chunks

juice of ½ orange

2 tsp chipotle paste

125g tinned kidney beans,
drained and rinsed

2 tortilla wraps

4 cherry tomatoes, halved

large handful of shredded
iceberg lettuce or similar

TUNA BURRITO

Nothing beats a giant burrito after a workout and this one with tuna steak won't disappoint. It's a big-boy portion so you'll need two tortillas to fit it all in.

METHOD

Melt the coconut oil in a large frying pan over a medium to high heat. Add the spring onions, garlic and tuna. Stir-fry for 2 minutes until you are happy the spring onions and garlic are cooked; the tuna will take care of itself.

Reduce the heat to medium, squeeze in the orange juice and then dollop in the chipotle paste. Give everything a good stir.

Tip in the kidney beans and cook for a further minute, just long enough for the beans to warm through.

Chuck the tortillas in the microwave for a few seconds, then divide the tuna mix between them, trying to stay in a central line. Top with the tomatoes and shredded lettuce, then roll them up.

Save these for later by covering with tin foil and keeping in the fridge until you're ready to eat.

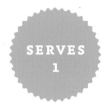

POST-WORKOUT
INGREDIENTS

½ tbsp coconut oil
1 rasher of smoked back bacon,
   trimmed of visible fat and
   sliced into 1cm strips
2 spring onions, finely sliced
1 clove garlic, finely chopped
1 x 240g skinless chicken
   breast fillet, sliced into 1cm
   strips
100g fresh spaghetti
1 egg yolk
juice of ½ lemon
½ tsp Dijon mustard
salt and pepper
1 tbsp chopped parsley

★ Serve with a fresh
green salad.

CHICKEN CARBONARA

I've only gone and made a carbonara sauce without dairy.
It's still creamy but I've cheated a bit.

METHOD

Put a saucepan of water on to boil.

Melt the coconut oil in a large frying pan over a medium to
high heat. Add the bacon, spring onions and garlic and stir-fry
for 1 minute.

Add the chicken, toss together with the other ingredients and
stir-fry for about 6 minutes, or until you are happy the chicken
is cooked through. Check by slicing into one of the larger
pieces to make sure the meat is white all the way through, with
no raw pink bits left.

When the water has come to the boil, drop in the spaghetti and
simmer for 2 minutes (or according to the packet instructions).

While the pasta is cooking, whisk the egg yolk with the lemon
juice and mustard until smooth. Just before draining the
pasta, spoon about 2 tablespoons of the hot, starchy cooking
liquid into the egg yolk mixture, whisking it until smooth.

Drain the pasta in a colander, give it a little shake and tip it
into the pan with the chicken. Pour in the egg yolk mix and
combine over a medium to low heat. The residual heat
will thicken the egg yolk sauce to become thick and velvety.

Season with salt and pepper, mix in the chopped parsley and
serve up the impossibly creamy, no-cream carbonara.

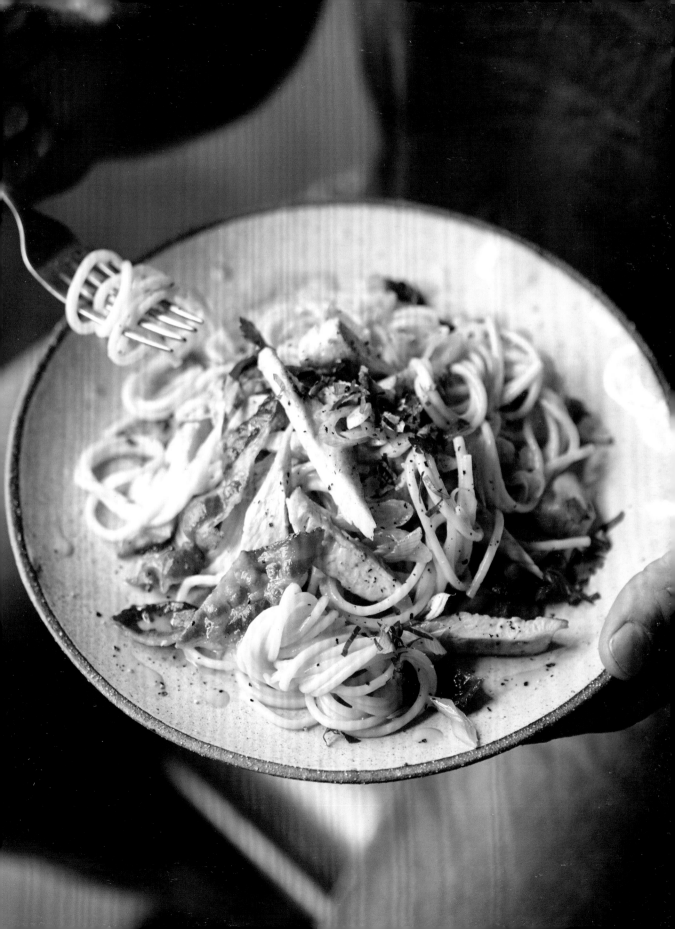

CHICKEN FAJITA FRIED RICE

POST-WORKOUT
MAKE AHEAD
INGREDIENTS

1 red onion, halved
4 cherry tomatoes, chopped
juice of 1 lime
½ tbsp coconut oil
¼ red pepper, de-seeded and
  finely sliced
3 baby sweetcorn, sliced in
  half on an angle
1 red chilli, de-seeded and
  finely sliced
1 x 240g skinless chicken
  breast fillet, sliced into 1cm
  strips
1 tsp ground cumin
1 tsp dried oregano
1 tsp smoked paprika
250g pre-cooked rice
handful of coriander, roughly
  chopped

Sometimes when I get in from the gym I can't be bothered
to mess about and want to eat right away. This is one of those
one-pot, no-hassle meals in true Lean in 15 style – quick,
simple and tasty!

METHOD

Dice one half of the onion and put it into a bowl. Slice the
other half roughly into 5 thin wedges. Add the tomatoes to
the bowl with the diced onion, squeeze over half of the lime
juice and leave to sit.

Melt the coconut oil in a large frying pan or wok over a medium
to high heat. Chuck in the onion wedges, red pepper and baby
sweetcorn and stir-fry for 2 minutes.

Now add the chilli and chicken and continue to stir-fry for
about 4 minutes, by which time the chicken should be pretty
much cooked through.

Stir in the cumin, oregano and smoked paprika and add the
rice, crumbling it between your fingers as you drop it in, then
pour in 2 tablespoons of water straight after. The water will
steam up and help finish cooking the ingredients as well as
separating the rice grains.

Give the whole lot a couple more tosses in the pan, to make
sure the rice is warmed through and the chicken fully cooked.
Check by slicing into one of the larger pieces to make sure the
meat is white all the way through, with no raw pink bits left.

Take the pan off the heat, stir half of the coriander through
the cooked rice and half through the onion, tomato and lime
mix, then serve everything up with the remaining lime juice
to squeeze over the rice.

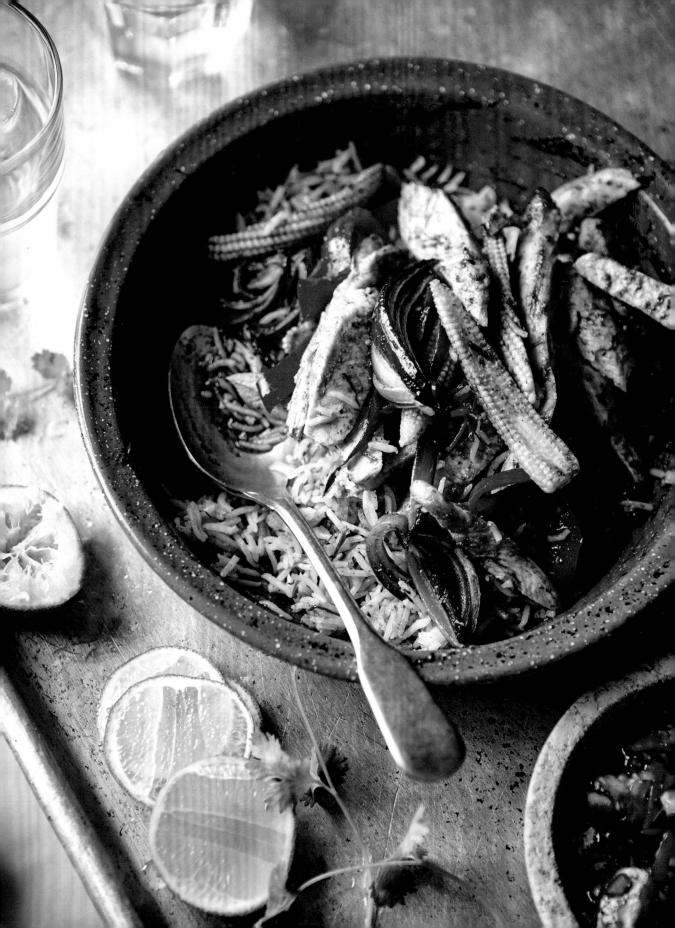

CHORIZO, TURKEY AND SWEET POTATO HASH

SERVES 1

POST-WORKOUT INGREDIENTS

1 sweet potato, peeled and roughly chopped into 2cm chunks

½ tbsp coconut oil

½ red onion, diced

large handful of kale

30g chorizo, chopped into 1cm pieces

1 x 240g skinless turkey breast fillet, sliced into 1cm strips

½ tsp ground cumin

½ tsp cayenne pepper (more if you like it spicy)

80g tinned sweetcorn, drained

1 red chilli, de-seeded and finely sliced

1 tbsp reduced-fat Greek yoghurt, to serve

handful of coriander, roughly chopped – optional

Love it or hate it, you can't deny that the microwave is an incredible invention. It's the machine that gives us back time and means we don't have to stand there like a plonker watching potatoes boil. This recipe has chorizo, too, so you know it's gonna be a winner.

METHOD

Place the sweet potato in a microwaveable dish and zap at 900w for 4 minutes. Leave to rest for 2 minutes and then zap for a further 4 minutes. Leave them to sit until ready to use.

Meanwhile, melt the coconut oil in a large frying pan over a medium to high heat. Add the onion, kale and chorizo and fry, stirring regularly, for about 3 minutes, by which time the vegetables will have softened.

Crank up the heat to maximum and slide in the turkey, tossing it in the pan with the other ingredients. Stir-fry over the high heat for about 3 minutes, or until the turkey is nearly done. Sprinkle in the cumin and cayenne pepper and fry, stirring constantly, for 30 seconds.

Tumble in the sweetcorn and the microwaved sweet potato and continue to fry for a further 2–3 minutes, or until you are certain the turkey is totally cooked through. Check by slicing into one of the larger pieces to make sure the meat is white all the way through, with no raw pink bits left. If you're worried that the pan is drying out or the spices are burning, add a splash of water, which will steam up and help everything cook through.

Slide your sunshine hash onto a plate and scatter with the fiery chilli. Serve with a dollop of cooling yoghurt and a sprinkling of chopped coriander, if using.

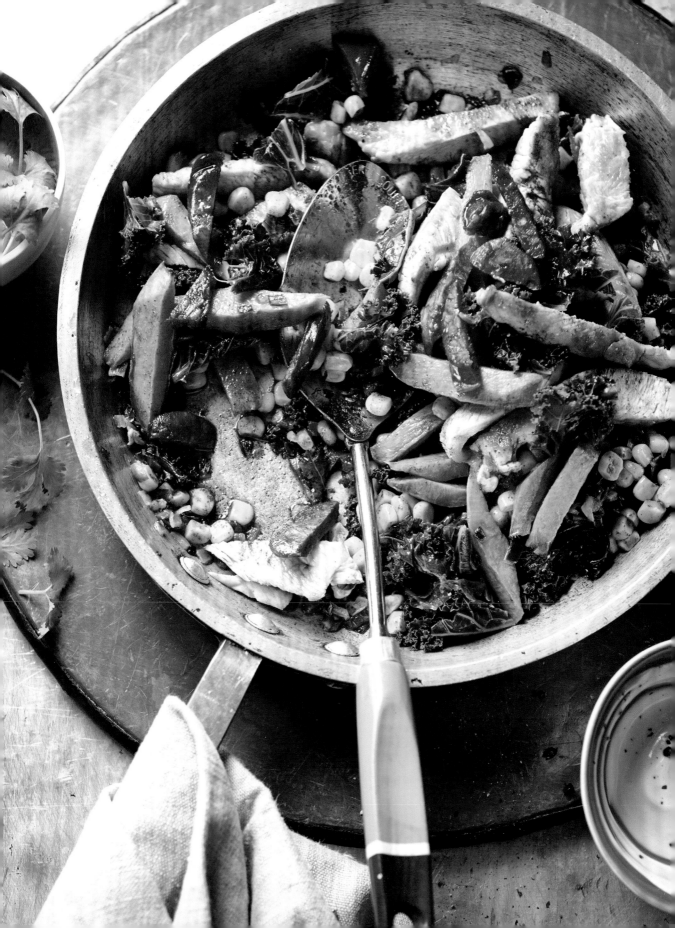

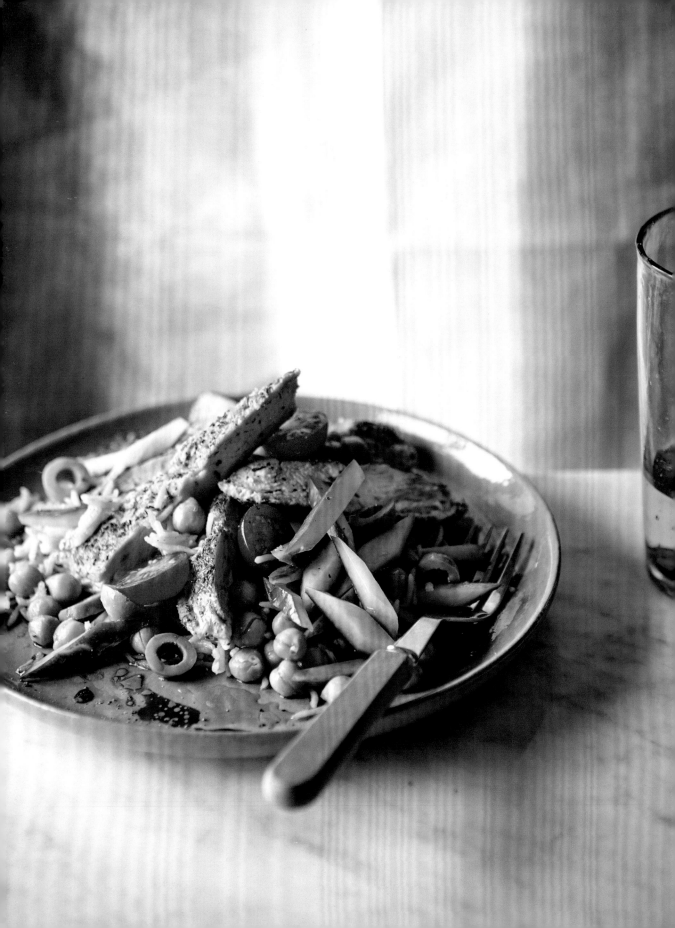

RICE, CHICKPEAS, CUCUMBERS AND CHICKEN

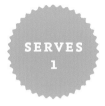

SERVES 1

POST-WORKOUT
MAKE AHEAD
INGREDIENTS

1 x 200g skinless chicken
  breast fillet
1½ tsp dried oregano
salt and pepper
100g pre-cooked rice
125g tinned chickpeas, drained
  and rinsed
½ tbsp olive oil
2 tsp balsamic vinegar
¼ cucumber, de-seeded and
  chopped into 2cm chunks
3 cherry tomatoes, halved
5 pitted green olives
handful of mint, leaves only

★ Serve with a fresh
green salad.

Okay, I admit it, this is a recipe that came about from me raiding my fridge for leftovers late one night. Odd combo but it really works, with the dressing and fresh mint bringing everything together.

METHOD

Preheat your grill to maximum.

Place the chicken between two pieces of cling film or baking parchment on a chopping board. Using a rolling pin, meat mallet or any other blunt instrument, bash the chicken until it is about 1cm thick all over.

Sprinkle the chicken with the oregano and a generous amount of salt and pepper, lay it on a grill pan and slide under the hot grill. Cook for 6 minutes on each side, or until you are sure the chicken is fully cooked. Check by slicing into a thicker part to make sure the meat is white all the way through, with no raw pink bits left.

While the chicken is cooking, mix together the rice and chickpeas and heat in the microwave just long enough for the ingredients to warm through.

Mix together the olive oil and balsamic vinegar in a bowl and add the cucumber and cherry tomatoes.

When the rice and chickpeas are hot, take them out of the microwave, add the olives and then combine with the cucumber and cherry tomatoes.

Plate up the rice and chickpea salad, top with the chicken and then scatter over the mint leaves.

SAUSAGE AND MUSHROOM PENNE PASTA

POST-WORKOUT

INGREDIENTS

½ tbsp coconut oil

½ red onion, diced

3 chestnut mushrooms, roughly quartered

4 chicken sausages (about 200g), chopped into 3cm chunks

100g fresh penne

4 midget trees (tender-stem broccoli), any bigger stalks sliced in half lengthways

1 jarred red pepper, drained and thinly sliced

5 pitted black olives, halved

salt and pepper

I'm not even going to introduce this recipe. It doesn't need it. I'm just going to let the picture talk. I can guarantee this is a recipe you'll be cracking out more than once a week.

METHOD

Put a saucepan of water on to boil.

Melt the coconut oil in a large frying pan over a medium to high heat. Chuck in the onion, mushrooms and sausage chunks. Fry the whole lot together, stirring every now and then, for about 5 minutes, or until the sausages are pretty much cooked through.

When the water comes to the boil, drop in the penne and midget trees and simmer for about 2 minutes (or according to the pasta packet instructions). The trees and penne should be cooked in about the same time. When they're done, drain in a colander and leave to one side.

Add the red pepper to the sausage mixture and toss the whole lot together. Crank up the heat a little and pour in about 2 tablespoons of water, which should steam up and evaporate pretty quickly – this will help to ensure the sausages are cooked through. Check by slicing into one of the larger pieces to make sure there are no raw pink bits left.

When you are happy the sausages are fully cooked, tumble in the olives and the drained pasta and trees. Give it all one final toss together and then serve up with a sprinkle of salt and pepper.

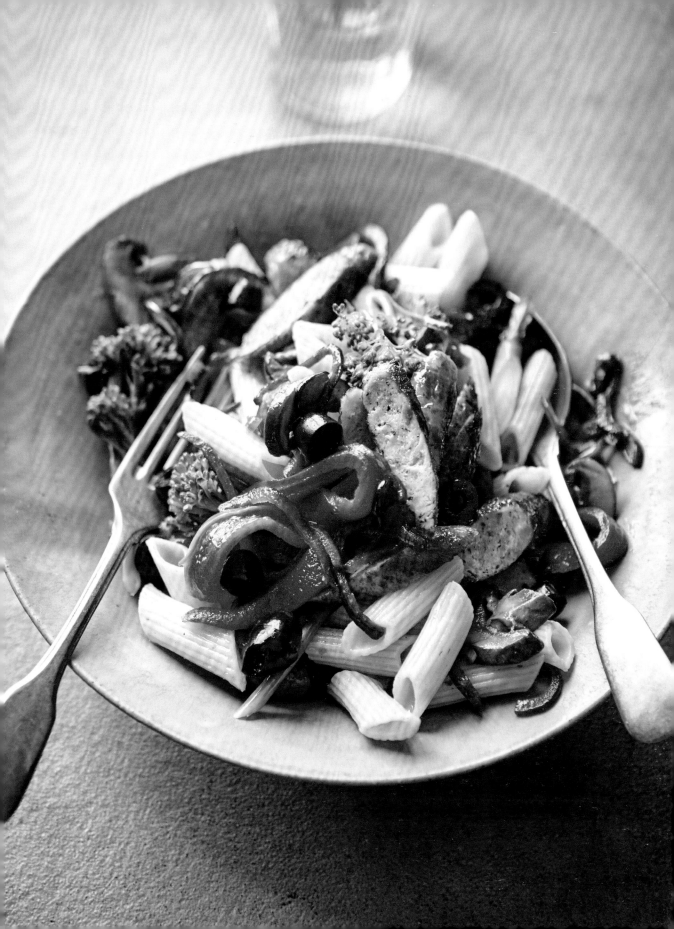

CHICKEN AND PRAWN PAPRIKA NOODLES

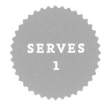

SERVES 1

POST-WORKOUT

INGREDIENTS

½ tbsp coconut oil

1 x 120g skinless chicken breast fillet, sliced into 1cm strips

2 spring onions, finely sliced

1 clove garlic, finely chopped

4 cherry tomatoes, halved

4 midget trees (tender-stem broccoli), any bigger stalks sliced in half lengthways

6 raw king prawns, peeled

2 tsp sweet smoked paprika

250g 'straight to wok' egg noodles

juice of 1 lime

1 red chilli, de-seeded and sliced – optional

It might sound like a strange mix having prawns and chicken in the same dish but trust me, it works. This is one of the easiest meals when you're in a rush to refuel after a workout.

METHOD

Melt the coconut oil in a large frying pan over a high heat. Add the chicken and stir-fry for 2 minutes.

Chuck in the spring onions, garlic, cherry tomatoes, midget trees and prawns. Stir-fry the whole lot together over the high heat for about 3 minutes – don't chicken out and reduce the heat.

Sprinkle in the smoked paprika and toss to coat the ingredients in the pan. Add the noodles, breaking up the clumps with your fingers as you drop them in. Pour in about 2 tablespoons of water, which will steam up and help cook through the noodles and the chicken. Check by slicing into one of the larger pieces to make sure the meat is white all the way through, with no raw pink bits left.

When you are sure the chicken is fully cooked, remove the pan from the heat and squeeze in the lime juice.

Plate up the noodles and top with red chilli, if using.

SWEET AND SOUR CHICKEN WITH RICE

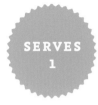

POST-WORKOUT INGREDIENTS

½ tbsp coconut oil

¼ red pepper, de-seeded and sliced into thin strips

½ red onion, sliced into 6 wedges

2 cloves garlic, roughly chopped

1 x 240g skinless chicken breast fillet, sliced into 1cm strips

4 cherry tomatoes, halved

100g fresh pineapple, chopped into 2cm chunks

1 tbsp honey

2 tbsp red wine vinegar

250g pre-cooked rice

1 tbsp light soy sauce

2 tsp sesame oil

handful of coriander, roughly chopped – optional

When I was young and my dad cooked dinner, he always used to make this. It was literally the only thing he could cook and I would sulk every time. Not because I don't like sweet and sour but because he used a nasty ready-made jar of sauce. Well, this one is the real deal because the sauce is homemade and is how it should taste. #Decent.

METHOD

Melt the coconut oil in a large frying pan or wok over a high heat. Add the red pepper, onion and garlic and stir-fry for 1 minute.

Chuck in the chicken, tomatoes and pineapple and stir-fry for a further 2 minutes, by which time the chicken should be almost cooked through.

Reduce the heat a little and pour in the honey and vinegar (watch yourself, as the steaming vinegar can be pretty intoxicating). Bring the whole lot to a simmer and cook like this for about 2 minutes, or until you are sure the chicken is fully cooked through and the sauce has thickened a little. Check the chicken is cooked by slicing into one of the larger pieces to make sure the meat is white all the way through, with no raw pink bits left.

While the chicken is cooking, ping the rice in the microwave, following the packet instructions.

Take the chicken off the heat and stir through the soy sauce, sesame oil and coriander, if using. Serve up the rice topped with the tasty sweet and sour chicken.

SPICED PRAWNS AND POTATOES

All hail the microwave – the king of quick carbs. It makes a Lean in 15 life so much easier. This dish is simple but satisfying.

POST-WORKOUT INGREDIENTS

1 large potato, chopped into 2cm cubes
½ tbsp coconut oil
½ red onion, diced
2 cloves garlic, finely chopped
¼ courgette, chopped into 2cm pieces
¼ red pepper, de-seeded and sliced into 1cm strips
1 egg
180g raw prawns, peeled
2 tsp smoked paprika
1 tsp turmeric
large handful of baby spinach leaves
juice of 1 lemon

METHOD

Zap the potato cubes in the microwave for 4 minutes, leave to rest for 1 minute and then blast for a further 3 minutes. Leave the potato in the microwave for now. Put a saucepan of water on to boil.

Meanwhile, melt half of the coconut oil in a frying pan over a medium to high heat. Chuck in the onion, garlic, courgette and red pepper and stir-fry for 2 minutes.

You will have to wait a little for the potato to finish cooking, so this is a good time to poach the egg, carefully cracking it into the hot water and reducing the heat until the water is just 'burping'. Cook the egg for about 4 minutes for a runny yolk, then carefully lift it out with a slotted spoon and drain on kitchen roll.

As soon as the spud is ready, add it to the frying pan along with the prawns. Crank the heat up to maximum and fry, stirring occasionally.

When the prawns are pretty much cooked through – their raw grey colour will turn pink – reduce the heat to medium and sprinkle in the spices, tossing to coat the ingredients in the pan. Pour in 1 tablespoon of water to prevent any burning.

Stir the baby spinach through the mixture, turn off the heat and let the leaves wilt in the residual heat.

Plate up the spiced prawns and spud mix and squeeze over a little lemon juice. Finish by crowning with your perfectly poached egg.

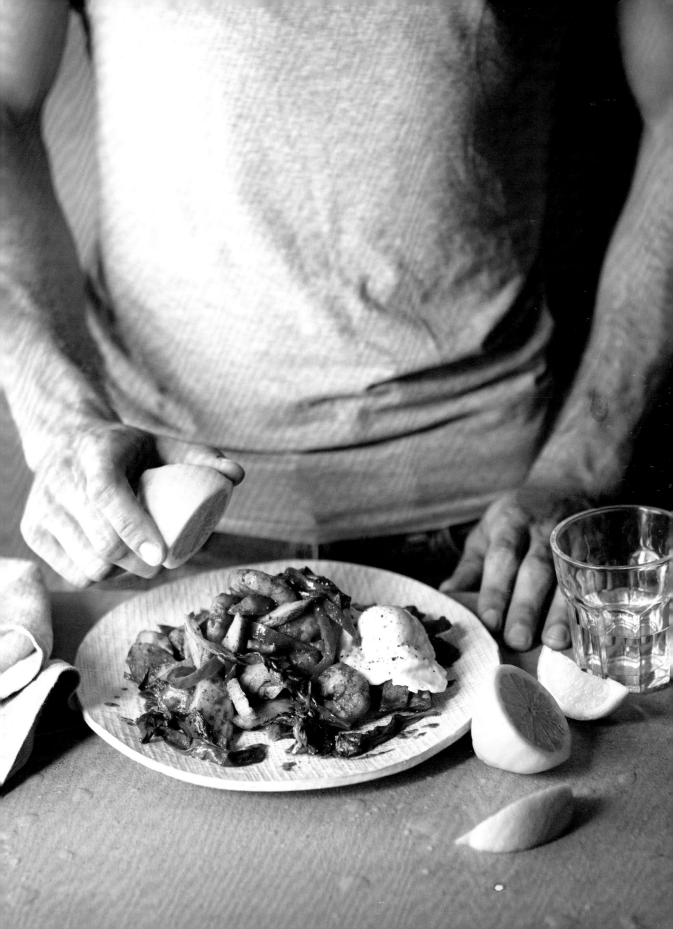

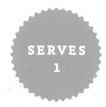

SERVES 1

SMOKY JOE BURGER AND WEDGES

Another burger recipe? Guilteeee! Sorry, but you know I'm a burger lover. This one with sweet potato wedges is probably one of my all-time favourite post-workout meals.

POST-WORKOUT INGREDIENTS

1 large sweet potato, sliced into 6 wedges
240g lean beef mince
2 tsp smoked paprika, plus a little extra for dusting
2 tsp onion granules
1 tsp salt, plus extra for sprinkling
¼ red onion, finely diced
½ tbsp coconut oil
1 large burger bun
½ tbsp reduced-fat Greek yoghurt
a few lettuce leaves, to serve
1 tomato, sliced, to serve

METHOD

Preheat your grill to maximum.

Zap the sweet potato wedges in the microwave at 900w for 4 minutes, leave to rest for 2 minutes, then blast for a further 3 minutes. Leave them in the microwave until you're ready to use them.

Meanwhile, put the beef mince, paprika, onion granules, salt and onion in a bowl. Mix the ingredients together really well – working the meat helps it to bind without having to throw in eggs or breadcrumbs.

Shape the mixture into one large patty about 1.5cm thick, lay it straight onto a baking tray and slide under the grill. Cook the burger for about 5 minutes on the first side, flip, then grill for 4 minutes on the second side. Switch off the grill but leave the burger to rest in the residual heat until you're ready to serve.

Melt the coconut oil in a frying pan over a high heat. Carefully slide in the zapped potato wedges and fry for about 2 minutes, or until lightly browned all over. Drain off any excess fat on a clean piece of kitchen roll, then sprinkle the wedges with salt and a little smoked paprika.

When you're ready to eat, plate up the wedges and cut the bun in half. Spread with a thin layer of yoghurt, then add the lettuce and sliced tomato, top with your burger, stick the lid on and get both hands involved.

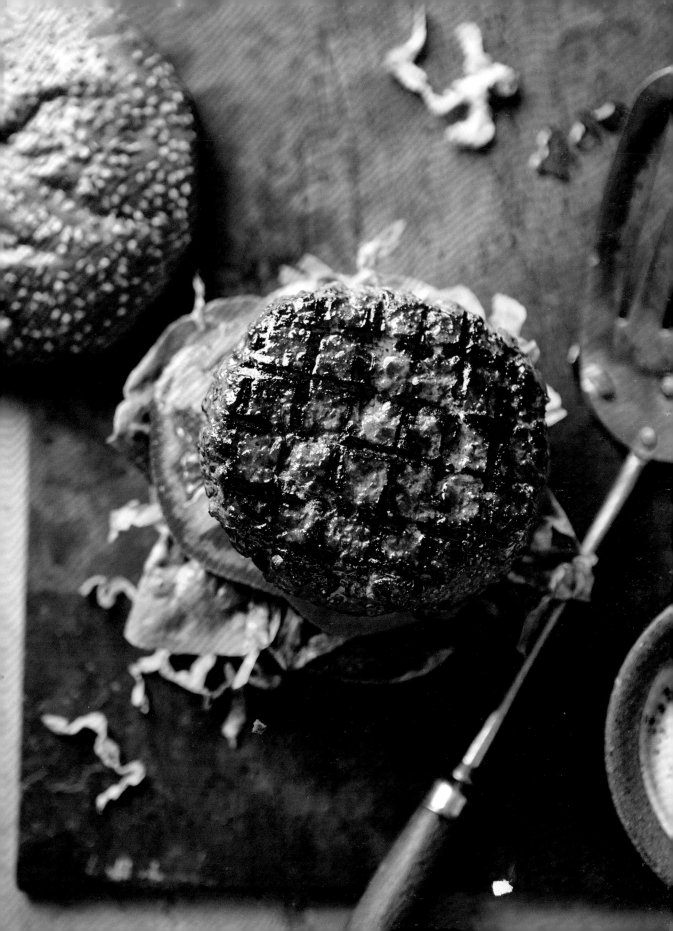

CHICKEN ORZO WITH HERBS AND LEMON

SERVES 1

POST-WORKOUT
INGREDIENTS

350ml chicken stock
½ tbsp coconut oil
1 clove garlic, roughly chopped
2 spring onions, finely sliced
1 x 250g skinless chicken
  breast fillet, sliced into 1cm
  strips
80g dried orzo
handful each of basil, chives
  and parsley
50g frozen peas
1 lemon
black pepper

Never had orzo before? Time to give it a go. It cooks like pasta and looks like rice. When you combine it with all these fresh herbs you've got yourself a real winner.

METHOD

Pour the stock into a small pan and put it on to boil over a high heat.

Melt the coconut oil in a large saucepan over a medium to high heat. Add the garlic and spring onions and fry for 1 minute before sliding in the chicken. Crank up the heat to maximum and stir all the ingredients together for about 2 minutes.

Tip in the orzo and pour in the hot stock (it should be pretty much boiling by this time). Bring the stock quickly up to the boil then clamp a lid on the pan and simmer for 10 minutes, or until the pasta is tender. It will probably be necessary to remove the lid and give the pasta a couple of stirs during the cooking time.

While the orzo is cooking, place all the herbs on your chopping board and chop them roughly into small pieces.

When the 10 minutes are up, remove the lid from the pasta and stir through the peas, cooking them for about 30 seconds, or until they are warmed through. The orzo should have absorbed much of the moisture and become thick and saucy.

Stir the chopped herbs through the cooked pasta and chicken and finish by squeezing in some lemon juice and grated zest, with a pinch of black pepper.

Serve up and get stuck in.

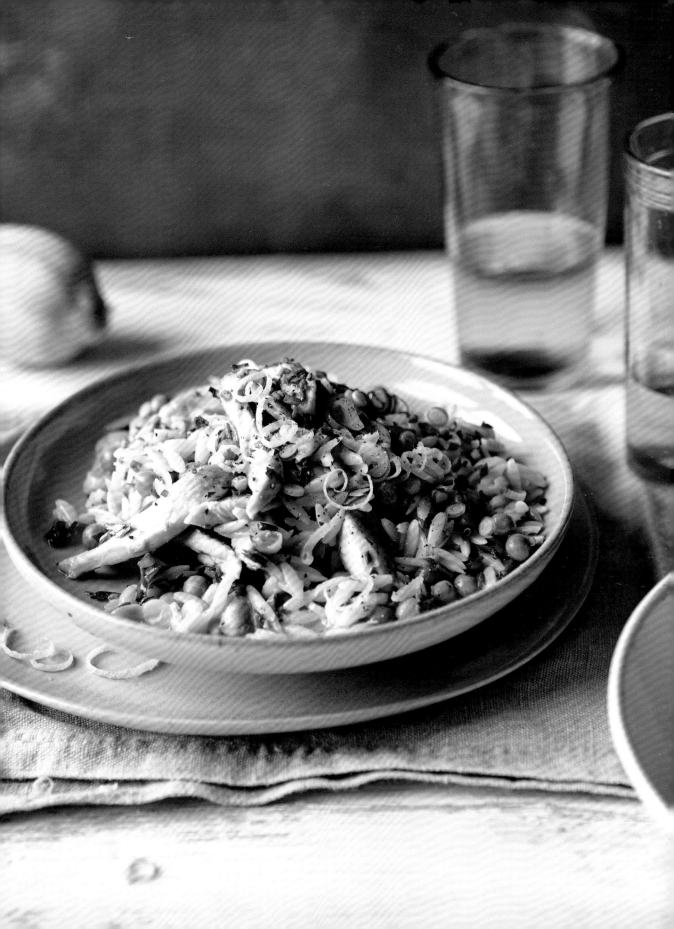

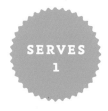

POST-WORKOUT
MAKE AHEAD
GOOD TO FREEZE
INGREDIENTS

½ tbsp coconut oil
2 spring onions, finely sliced
1 clove garlic, finely chopped
240g turkey mince
1 tbsp tomato puree
1 tsp caster sugar
1 tsp dried oregano
2 tbsp balsamic or red wine
   vinegar
200g tinned chopped
   tomatoes
90g fresh pasta sheets, cut in
   half (about 3 sheets)
handful of basil leaves

15-MINUTE TURKEY LASAGNE

A lasagne in 15 minutes? Is he having a laugh? Well, it seems a bit crazy but actually, yes, it is possible when you follow this recipe and take a few shortcuts. But don't be fooled – even though this dish is quick, it's not missing out on flavour.

METHOD

Put a saucepan of water on to boil.

Melt the coconut oil in a large frying pan over a high heat. Add the spring onions, garlic and turkey mince. Fry the ingredients for about 2 minutes, stirring only occasionally. After 2 minutes, get your wooden spoon stuck in to help break up the large chunks of mince.

Continue frying and breaking up the mince until there are no large chunks left. Squeeze in the tomato puree and sprinkle in the sugar and oregano. Keep on frying and stirring over the high heat for 1 minute and then pour in the vinegar, letting it bubble up and evaporate to almost nothing.

Now tip in the chopped tomatoes and bring the whole lot to a gentle simmer. Cook like this for about 2–3 minutes, or until you are certain the turkey mince is fully cooked through – all the meat should have turned from raw pink to cooked white.

While the mince is bubbling away, slide your lasagne sheets into the boiling water and simmer for about 5 minutes, or until just tender.

When you are sure the turkey is cooked, remove the pan from the heat.

To serve, I like to lay a sheet of cooked pasta on the base of my pasta bowl, top with mince and then repeat the layers until I've used up all my pasta and mince mix. Finish with a scattering of basil.

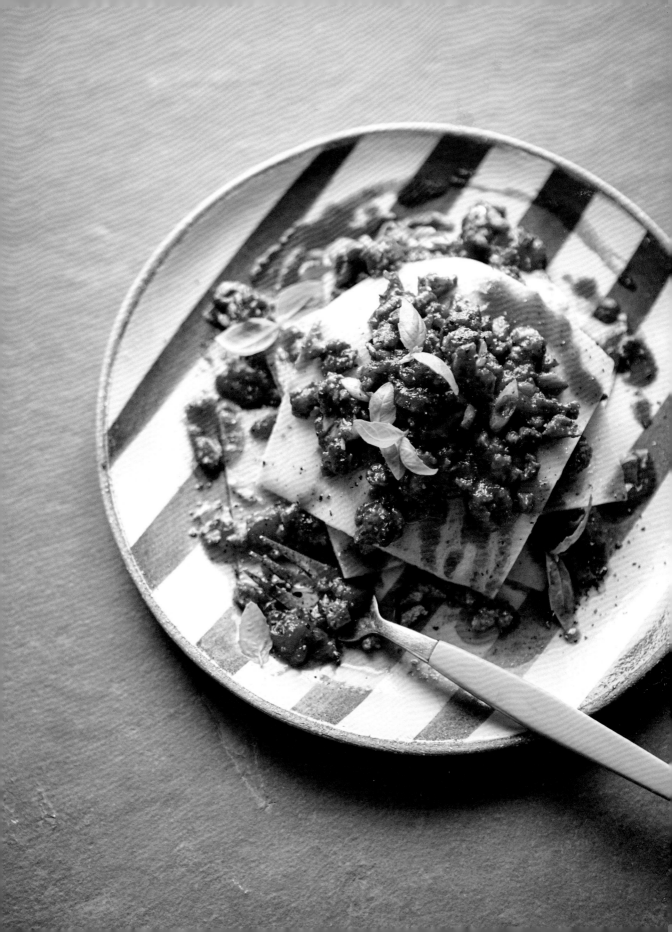

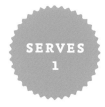

POST-WORKOUT
MAKE AHEAD
INGREDIENTS

½ tbsp tomato puree
3 tsp garam masala
1 tsp turmeric
2 cloves garlic, finely chopped
juice of 1 lemon
1 x 240g skinless chicken
  breast fillet, sliced into 1cm
  strips
½ tbsp coconut oil
¼ red onion, finely sliced
1 large baguette
2 tbsp mango chutney
handful of shredded lettuce
handful of coriander

CHICKEN TIKKA BAGUETTE

What's not to like about this? Forget about ordering a greasy takeaway. This homemade chicken tikka in a massive baguette is a dream and it's the perfect post-workout refuel meal. You're going to want to eat this one again and again.

METHOD

Squeeze the tomato puree into a bowl and sprinkle in the garam masala and turmeric. Add the garlic and lemon juice and mix the whole lot together until it forms a paste. Plonk the chicken strips into the mix and stir to coat as much of the meat as possible.

Melt the coconut oil in a large frying pan over a medium to high heat. Add the onion and stir-fry for 2 minutes. Chuck in the marinated chicken and toss together with the onion.

Pour in about 2 tablespoons of water, and reduce the heat a little so that the chicken is gently simmering away. Cook the chicken like this for about 8 minutes, or until you are sure it is cooked through. Check by slicing into one of the larger pieces to make sure the meat is white all the way through, with no raw pink bits left.

While the chicken is cooking, slice open the baguette and spread the mango chutney all over. When the chicken is cooked, scoop it into the baguette, top with the shredded lettuce and scatter over a load of coriander.

Grab a napkin as I'm pretty sure this is going to get messy.

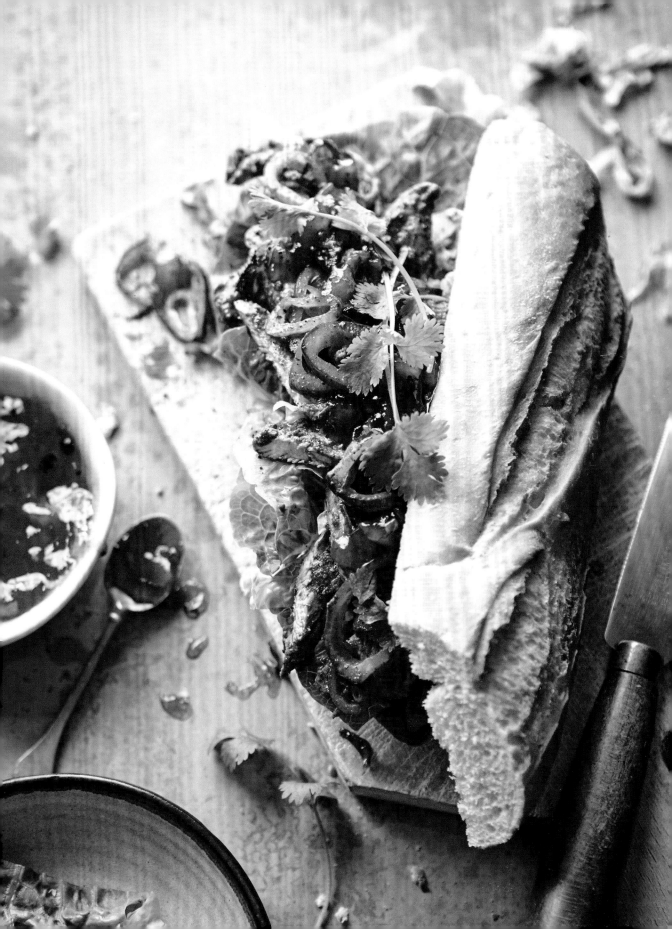

POST-WORKOUT
MAKE AHEAD
INGREDIENTS

½ tbsp coconut oil
2 spring onions, finely sliced
2cm ginger, finely diced
1 lemongrass stalk, tender
  white part only, finely sliced
1 clove garlic, finely chopped
1 x 240g sirloin steak, trimmed
  of visible fat and sliced into
  1cm strips
40g mange tout or green
  beans
4 baby sweetcorn, halved
250g 'straight to wok' egg
  noodles
2 tsp fish sauce
juice of 1 lime
handful of coriander, roughly
  chopped
1 red chilli, finely sliced

LEMONGRASS AND GINGER BEEF NOODLES

All done in one pan with no fuss – a fiery little number which
is a true Lean in 15 recipe and ideal for a lunch box at work,
eaten either hot or cold. It tastes incredible with chicken too,
so feel free to mix it up.

METHOD

Melt the coconut oil in a large frying pan or wok over a high
heat. Add the spring onions, ginger, lemongrass and garlic and
stir-fry for 1 minute.

Add the steak and continue stir-frying over the high heat for
2 minutes, or until the beef is lightly coloured all over.

Chuck in the mange tout or green beans and the baby sweetcorn
and toss to mix with the rest of the ingredients. Add the noodles
followed quickly by 2 tablespoons of water, which will steam
up to help cook the vegetables and warm the noodles.

Continue stir-frying for another 2 minutes, or until you are
happy the noodles are heated through and the steak is cooked –
I like mine just a little pink on the inside.

Take the pan off the heat and stir through the fish sauce
and lime juice.

Serve up the noodles topped with a sprinkling of chopped
coriander and the sliced red chilli for a little extra heat.

GREEN CHILLI CHICKEN TAGLIATELLE

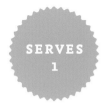

POST-WORKOUT INGREDIENTS

½ tbsp coconut oil
1 large green chilli, de-seeded and thinly sliced
1 clove garlic, finely chopped
2 spring onions, finely sliced
1 x 240g skinless chicken breast fillet, sliced into 1cm strips
100g fresh tagliatelle
large handful of kale, stalks removed
5 pitted green olives, halved
salt and pepper

If you love pasta then this one is defo for you. It's a recipe inspired by my Italian nan. She always used to try to make me eat olives as a kid and I would hate it. But somewhere along the way I started to love them.

METHOD

Bring a large saucepan of water to the boil.

Melt the coconut oil in a large frying pan over a medium to high heat. Add the chilli, garlic and spring onions and stir-fry for 1 minute.

Slide in the chicken and crank up the heat to maximum. Stir-fry the chicken for about 6 minutes, or until you are happy it is cooked through. Check by slicing into one of the larger pieces to make sure the meat is white all the way through, with no raw pink bits left.

When the water has come to the boil, drop in the pasta. As soon as the water comes back up to the boil, chuck in the kale leaves (they will all wilt down). Simmer the pasta and kale until both are tender – about 2 minutes. Drain in a colander, shaking off as much of the excess liquid as possible.

Add the olives to the pan with the chicken and then tip in the drained pasta and kale. Toss the whole lot together, adding a little salt and pepper.

Serve up your bright green pasta feast.

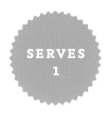

POST-WORKOUT
INGREDIENTS

½ tbsp coconut oil
½ red onion, diced
6 fennel seeds
½ fennel bulb, chopped into
   1cm pieces
1 celery stick, chopped into
   1cm pieces
1 tbsp tomato puree
juice of ½ orange
200g tinned chopped
   tomatoes
1 x 240g skinless cod fillet,
   chopped into large chunks
100g fresh tagliatelle
small handful of basil leaves
black pepper

COD
TAGLIATELLE

Hang on a minute. I thought pasta was a big no-no when trying to burn fat? Again, that's a myth. The body loves carbs after a big training session, so if you love pasta then go for it.

METHOD

Put a saucepan of water on to boil.

Melt the coconut oil in a large frying pan over a medium to high heat. Throw in the onion, fennel seeds, fennel and celery. Stir-fry for 3 minutes until the vegetables are just starting to soften.

Squeeze in the tomato puree, mix in with the rest of the ingredients and keep stir-frying for another minute.

Pour in the orange juice swiftly followed by the chopped tomatoes and give it all a good stir. Bring the whole lot to the boil and simmer for 1 minute. Drop in the cod and cook gently for about 3 minutes, or until you are happy that the fish is cooked through – you can check this by cutting into one of the thickest pieces to make sure it has turned from raw, pale flesh to cooked bright white.

Drop your tagliatelle into the boiling water and cook according to the packet instructions. Drain in a colander and plate up.

Spoon the cod and sauce over the pasta, and serve garnished with a little basil and black pepper.

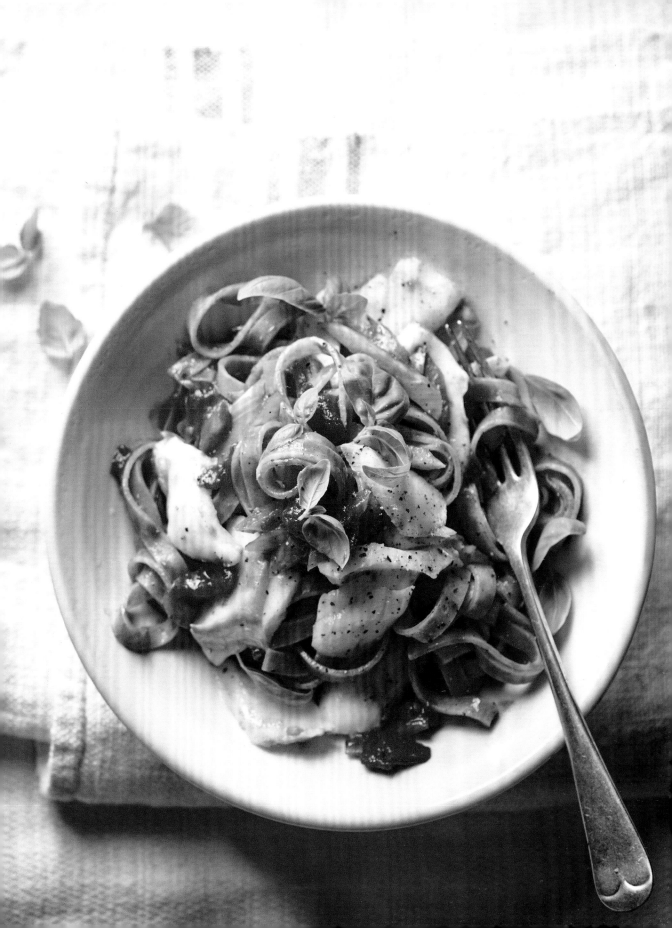

POST-WORKOUT
GOOD TO FREEZE
INGREDIENTS

1 large sweet potato, peeled
  and chopped into large
  chunks
½ tbsp coconut oil
3 spring onions, finely sliced
1 small carrot, grated
1 red chilli, de-seeded and
  finely sliced
240g lean beef mince
1 tbsp flour
50g frozen peas
150ml beef stock
3 tbsp Worcestershire sauce
salt and pepper

★ Serve with a pile of midget
trees (tender-stem
broccoli) and spinach or
green beans.

IN-A-HURRY COTTAGE PIE

I know you're probably thinking there's no way you can
cook a cottage pie in 15 minutes. But this is my version and
I've introduced a few shortcuts to make it possible.

METHOD

Blast the potato in the microwave for 4 minutes, rest for
2 minutes and then blast for a further 4 minutes. Leave in
the microwave for now.

Meanwhile, melt the coconut oil in a large frying pan over
a high heat. Throw in the spring onions, carrot and chilli and
fry for 30 seconds, stirring almost constantly.

Push the veg to the sides and plonk your mince right in the
middle of the pan. Leave it to brown on one side without
touching it for about 45 seconds. Then get stuck in with your
wooden spoon to break up the meat, making sure it's all cooked
through – don't even think about turning down the heat.

After 2–3 minutes the beef will have turned from pink to brown,
which means it's cooked. Sprinkle in the flour, stir to mix with
the rest of the ingredients and quickly follow with the peas and
beef stock. Now you can reduce the heat just a little and stir the
whole lot together until the sauce has thickened.

Remove the pan from the heat and stir through the Worcestershire
sauce. Spoon the mix onto a plate, give the sweet potato a quick
bash with a masher, adding a little salt and pepper along the way,
and then splodge over the cottage pie mix.

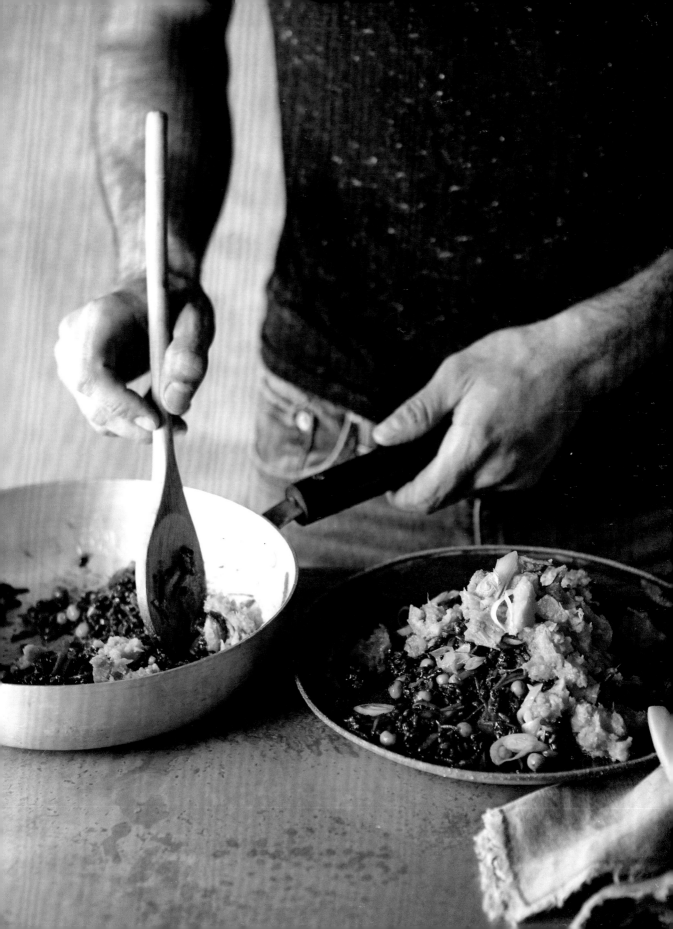

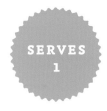

**SERVES
1**

INGREDIENTS

½ tbsp coconut oil

1 x 240g sirloin steak, trimmed
  of visible fat

salt and pepper

juice of 1 lime

1 tbsp fish sauce

2 tsp light soy sauce

½ tsp sesame oil

1 red chilli, finely chopped

2 spring onions, finely sliced

¼ red pepper, de-seeded and
  finely sliced

¼ cucumber, de-seeded and
  sliced into thin half-moons

½ carrot, thinly sliced

½ mango, roughly chopped
  into cubes or slices (about
  100g)

220g pre-cooked thin rice
  noodles

handful of coriander, roughly
  chopped

small handful of mint

THAI BEEF NOODLE SALAD

I love Thai food and whenever I travel to Thailand this salad is the first thing I order when I arrive. It's also a great lunch to prep the night before and take to work.

METHOD

Melt the coconut oil in a frying pan over a high heat. When it's really, really hot, season your steak and carefully lay it in the pan. Fry for 4 minutes on each side for medium rare, then leave it to rest until you're ready to eat.

While the steak is cooking, mix together the lime juice, fish sauce, soy sauce, sesame oil and chilli and set aside.

In a large bowl toss together all the remaining ingredients, then pour over the dressing and toss once more to coat them.

Slice up the steak, toss it in with the noodle salad, then pile it high and serve. Yum.

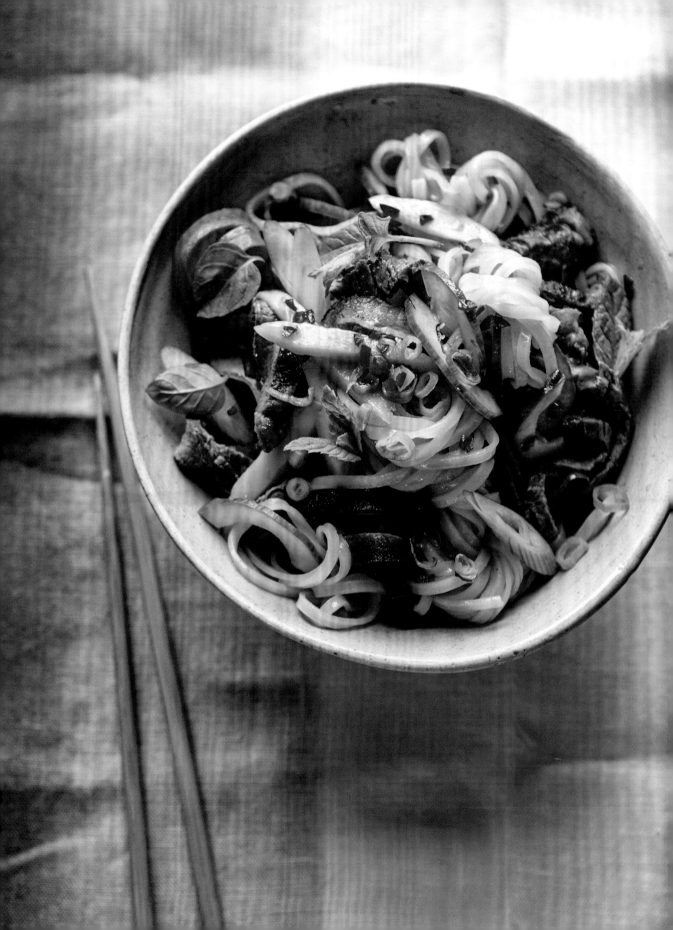

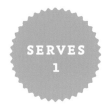

POST-WORKOUT
GOOD TO FREEZE
INGREDIENTS

1 sweet potato, peeled and
   chopped into 3cm chunks
½ tbsp coconut oil
½ red onion, diced
4 chicken sausages (roughly
   200g), chopped into large
   chunks
2 sprigs of thyme
1 bay leaf
1 celery stick, diced
½ courgette, diced
50g kale, stalks removed
125g tinned butter beans,
   drained and rinsed
300ml chicken stock

★ Serve with some crusty
bread and a pile of midget
trees (tender-stem broccoli).

SUPER-SPEEDY SAUSAGE STEW

Just because it's called a stew doesn't mean you have to wait
hours for it to cook. I've used the microwave to speed things up
here, but it still tastes amazing and is ready in 15 minutes, too.

METHOD

Zap the sweet potato in the microwave for 3 minutes, leave it
to rest for 2 minutes, then zap for another 3 minutes. Leave the
potato in the microwave for now.

Meanwhile, melt the coconut oil in a large saucepan over a
medium to high heat. Add the onion, sausages, thyme, bay
leaf, celery and courgette. Stir-fry for 4 minutes, then crank up
the heat to maximum. Add the kale leaves, butter beans and
stock and bring up to the boil.

Simmer the stew for 1 minute, then drop in the cooked sweet
potato, clamp on a lid and continue simmering for about
3 minutes, or until you are sure the sausages are fully cooked
through. Check by slicing into one of the larger pieces to make
sure the meat is white all the way through, with no raw pink
bits left.

Ladle the hearty stew into a bowl and, if it's been a particularly
tough workout, grab a piece of bread to dip in.

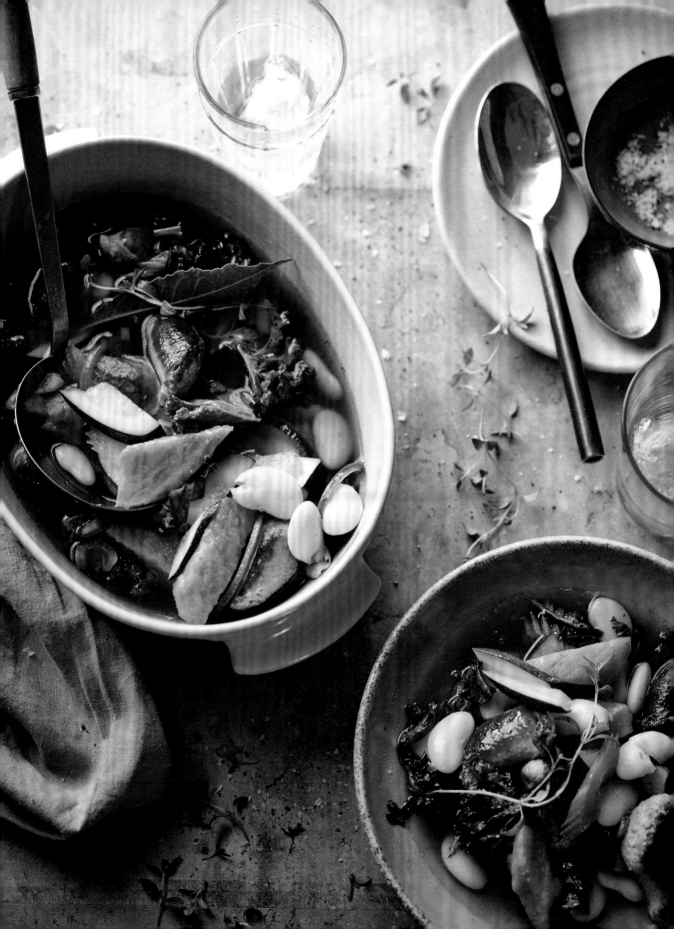

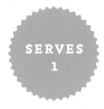

POST-WORKOUT
GOOD TO FREEZE
INGREDIENTS

200g pre-cooked puy lentils
½ tbsp coconut oil
½ carrot, diced
¼ leek, trimmed, washed and
  finely chopped
1 celery stick, diced
1 rasher of smoked back
  bacon, roughly chopped
1 tomato, roughly chopped
  into small pieces
2 sprigs of thyme
1 x 240g skinless cod fillet,
  chopped into 3cm chunks
75ml chicken or fish stock
1 tbsp chopped parsley
juice of ½ lemon
salt and pepper

ASIAN COD AND LENTILS

Lentils were always something I steered clear of because they take aaaages to prep, but now that you can pick up ready-cooked ones I'm a big fan. Speed is key when it comes to cooking and staying lean.

METHOD

Ping the lentils in the microwave according to the packet instructions. Leave to one side until ready to use.

Melt the coconut oil in a frying pan over a medium to high heat. Add the carrot, leek, celery and bacon and fry, stirring every now and then, for 2 minutes.

Add the tomato and thyme and fry for 1 minute, then add the cod and cook in with the other ingredients for about 1 minute.

Pour in the stock and bring up to the boil. Simmer the cod, turning the chunks a couple of times until they are cooked – you can check this by cutting into one of the thickest pieces to make sure it has turned from raw, pale flesh to cooked bright white. Tip the heated lentils into the pan and mix in.

When you are happy the cod is cooked, take the pan off the heat and stir through the parsley, lemon juice and a good pinch of salt and pepper.

Serve up and taste what's hot this year.

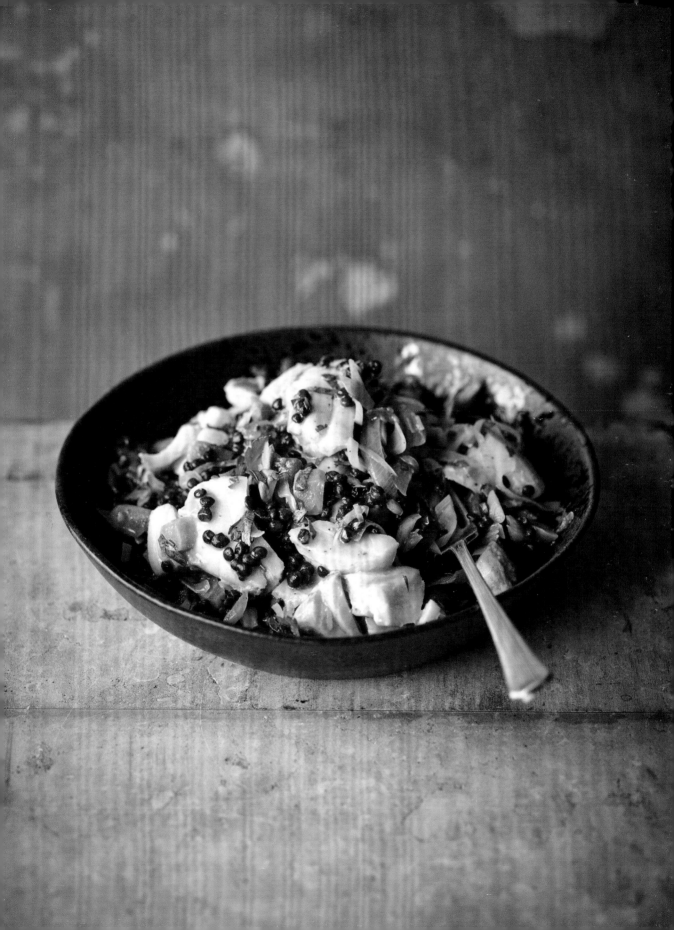

TURKEY, LEEK AND TARRAGON GNOCCHI

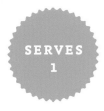

POST-WORKOUT
INGREDIENTS

½ tbsp coconut oil
¼ leek, trimmed, washed and
  finely sliced
40g kale, stalks removed
2 spring onions, finely sliced
4 chestnut mushrooms,
  sliced
1 x 240g skinless turkey breast
  fillet, sliced into 1cm strips
150g fresh gnocchi
handful of tarragon, leaves
  only, finely sliced
salt and pepper
juice of ½ lemon

Gnocchi is basically the love child of pasta and potato. It's such a satisfying carb source to eat after a workout. If you prefer to use chicken with this recipe, then go for it.

METHOD

Put a saucepan of water on to boil.

Melt the coconut oil in a large frying pan over a medium to high heat. Chuck in the leek, kale and spring onions and fry for 4–5 minutes, stirring regularly.

Increase the heat to maximum and add the mushrooms and turkey to the pan. Fry, stirring regularly, for about 4 minutes, or until you are happy the turkey is fully cooked. Check by slicing into one of the larger pieces to make sure the meat is white all the way through, with no raw pink bits left.

While the turkey is cooking, tip the gnocchi into the boiling water and cook according to the packet instructions.

When the gnocchi is cooked, drain in a colander and tip straight into the pan with the turkey. Turn off the heat, sprinkle in the tarragon along with a pinch of salt and pepper, and toss everything together.

Serve up with a refreshing squeeze of lemon.

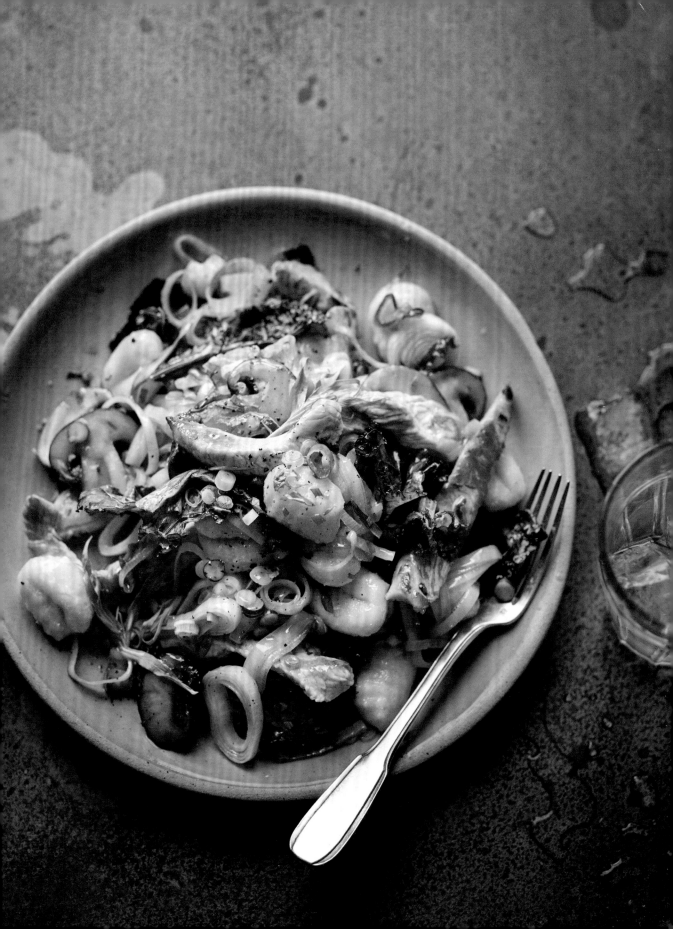

POST-WORKOUT
MAKE AHEAD

INGREDIENTS

1 x 240g skinless chicken
  breast fillet, sliced into 1cm
  strips
2 tsp tomato puree
juice of 1 lemon
salt and pepper
½ tbsp coconut oil
½ red onion, sliced
2 cloves garlic, finely chopped
2 tsp smoked paprika
1 tsp ground cumin
2 medium wholemeal pitta
  breads
large handful of shredded
  iceberg lettuce
6 cherry tomatoes, halved
½ cucumber, de-seeded,
  halved and sliced
reduced-fat Greek yoghurt,
  to serve
pickled chilli, to serve

CHICKEN SHISH

If, like me, you always end up ordering a chicken shish from the kebab shop when you're steam boat after a night out, you'll love this recipe. Keep it lean and try this healthier version when you're next craving a takeaway.

METHOD

Chuck the chicken into a small bowl and squeeze over the tomato puree and lemon juice along with a decent pinch of salt and pepper. Give the ingredients a good mix.

Melt the coconut oil in a frying pan over a medium to high heat. Add the onion and garlic and stir-fry for 2 minutes, or until the onion is just starting to soften.

Sprinkle in the paprika and cumin and cook for about 30 seconds, stirring constantly.

Crank up the heat to maximum and scrape in the chicken mixture. Stir-fry everything for about 2 minutes, or just long enough for the chicken to brown lightly. Pour in about 2 tablespoons of water, which will bubble up quickly. Reduce the heat to a simmer and cook for about 4 more minutes, or until you are happy the chicken is fully cooked. Check by slicing into one of the larger pieces to make sure the meat is white all the way through, with no raw pink bits left.

While the chicken is cooking, drop your pittas into a toaster and heat through.

Cut open your toasted pittas and spoon in the cooked chicken mixture. Stuff with as much crunchy lettuce, tomato and cucumber as you can, and finish with a drizzle of yoghurt and a hefty pickled chilli.

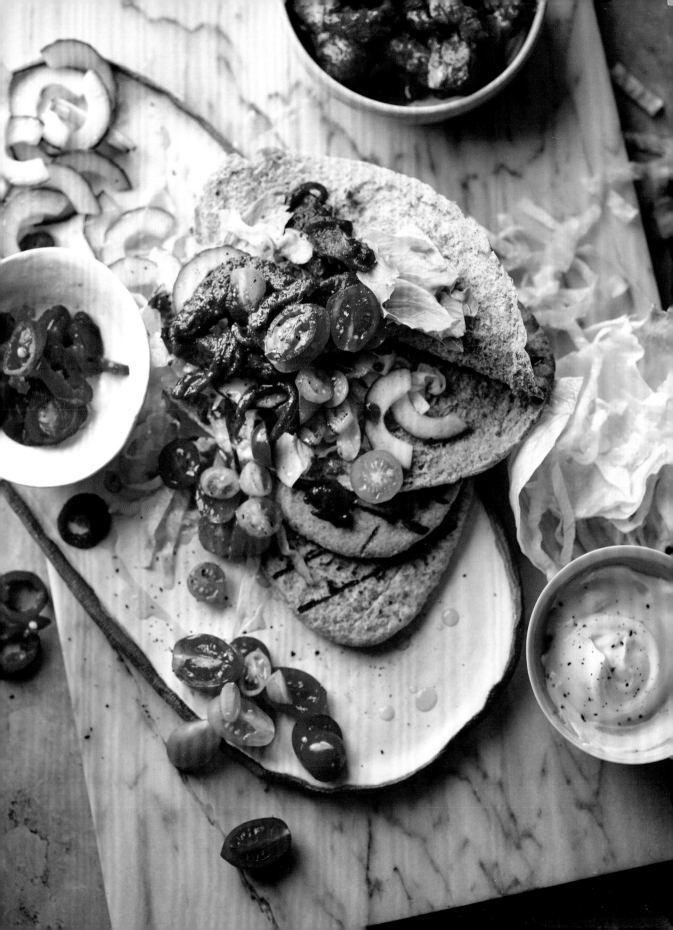

JEWELLED RICE WITH GRILLED LAMB

SERVES 1

POST-WORKOUT INGREDIENTS

240g lamb leg steaks (roughly 2 steaks)
½ tsp ground cumin
¼ tsp ground cinnamon
salt and pepper
250g pre-cooked rice
¼ cucumber, de-seeded and diced
1 celery stick, diced
1 jarred red pepper, drained and thinly sliced
2 spring onions, finely sliced
2 tsp balsamic vinegar
15g raisins
handful each of mint and parsley, roughly chopped
2 tbsp pomegranate seeds
juice of ½ lemon
drizzle of pomegranate molasses – optional

Okay, so pomegranate seeds and raisins may not be actual 'jewels' but they make the rice taste unreal and look pretty good, too, so I call this dish 'jewelled rice'. I think you'll love the flavours in this one.

METHOD

Preheat your grill to maximum.

Lay the lamb steaks on a baking tray, season with the cumin, cinnamon, salt and pepper and cook under the hot grill for 6 minutes, then flip over and cook for 4 minutes on the other side. Turn off the heat and leave the steaks to keep warm and rest until you're ready to serve.

Ping the rice in your microwave according to the packet instructions. When cooked, carefully tip the hot rice into a bowl, then add all the remaining ingredients (except for the lemon juice and pomegranate molasses) along with a decent pinch of salt and pepper. Mix everything together until well combined.

Pile the beautiful rice onto a plate and top with the sliced lamb steaks. Finish with a squeeze of lemon and a drizzle of pomegranate molasses, if using.

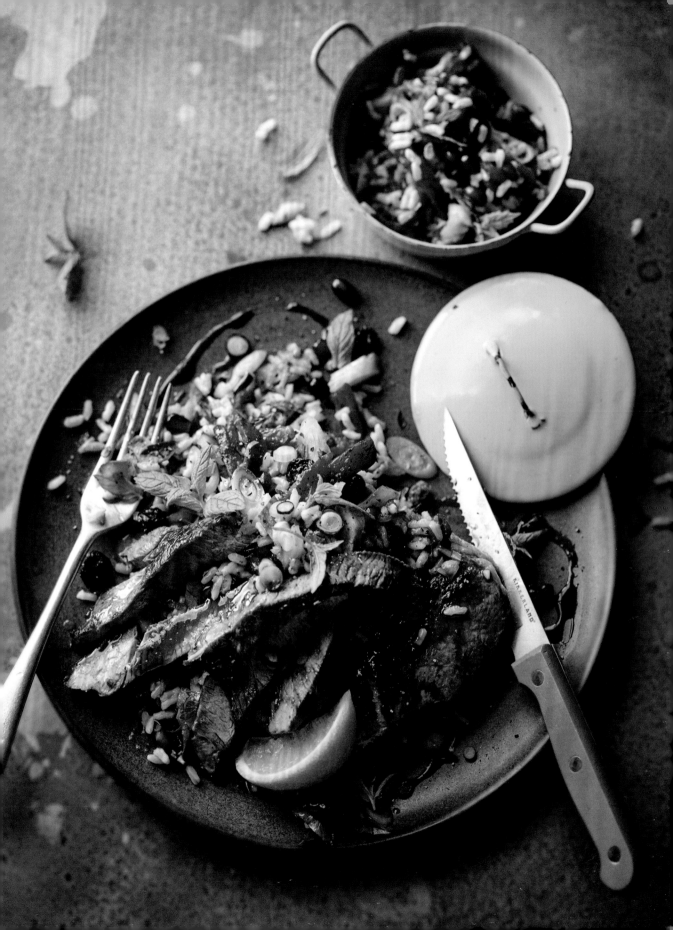

THAI-STYLE MIDGET TREE CHICKEN STIR-FRY

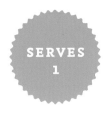

POST-WORKOUT
MAKE AHEAD

INGREDIENTS

1 tbsp coconut oil

3 spring onions, finely sliced

2cm ginger, finely chopped

handful of coriander, leaves
  and stalks separated

4 midget trees (tender-stem
  broccoli), any bigger stalks
  cut in half lengthways

1 lemongrass stalk, tender
  white part only, finely sliced

1 green chilli, finely sliced –
  remove the seeds if you don't
  like it hot

1 x 200g skinless chicken
  breast fillet, sliced into 1cm
  strips

250g pre-cooked egg noodles

1 egg

1 tbsp fish sauce

small handful of beansprouts

lime wedges, to serve

black pepper

Quick, easy and tasty – another classic Lean in 15 recipe.
Just in case you didn't know, midget trees is the name I've
given to broccoli.

METHOD

Melt half of the coconut oil in a large frying pan or wok over
a high heat. Chuck in the spring onions and ginger, then
roughly chop the coriander stalks and throw those in along
with the midget trees, lemongrass and chilli. Stir-fry the whole
lot for 1 minute and then add the chicken.

Stir-fry for about 5 more minutes, or until the chicken is pretty
much cooked through. Add the noodles, breaking up the
clumps with your fingers as you drop them in, quickly followed
by 2 tablespoons of water, which will steam up, helping the
noodles to warm through and ensuring the chicken is fully
cooked. Continue stir-frying until you are certain the chicken
is cooked through. Check by slicing into one of the larger
pieces to make sure the meat is white all the way through,
with no raw pink bits left.

Melt the remaining coconut oil in a small frying pan over a
medium to high heat and crack in the egg. Fry the egg to
your liking – I like a runny yolk and an almost crisp white for
this sort of dish.

When you are happy that all the stir-fried ingredients are cooked,
remove the pan from the heat. Roughly chop up the coriander
leaves and stir through the noodles along with the fish sauce.

Pile the noodles high on a plate, top with the beansprouts
and then lay the runny egg on top. Serve with wedges of lime
to squeeze over, along with a pinch of black pepper.

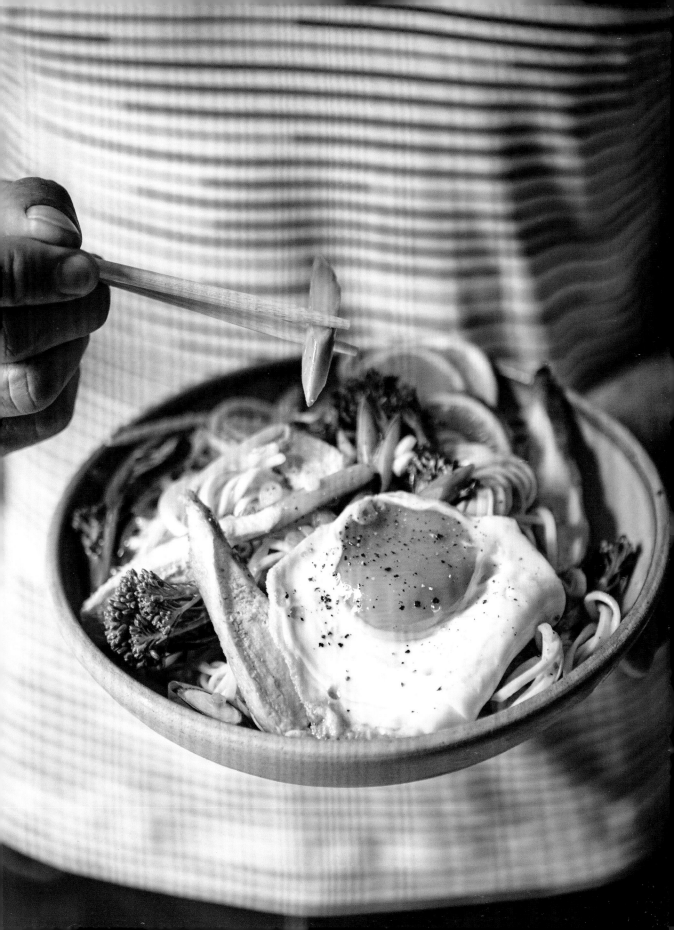

QUICK HERB AND TOMATO ORZOTTO

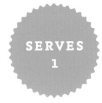

SERVES 1

INGREDIENTS

100g dried orzo
4 cherry tomatoes, on the vine
   if possible
salt and pepper
½ tbsp coconut oil
¼ leek, trimmed, washed and
   finely sliced
1 clove garlic, finely chopped
1 x 240g skinless chicken
   breast fillet, sliced into 1cm
   strips
1½ tbsp tomato puree
100ml chicken stock
handful each of basil, chives
   and parsley, roughly chopped
juice of ½ lemon

Okay, so I'm cheating a bit here as I'm not using risotto rice; I'm using orzo pasta. That's why I call it an 'orzotto'. It's quicker than risotto and in my opinion tastes better. #Win.

METHOD

Put a saucepan of water on to boil and preheat your grill to maximum.

As soon as the water comes to the boil, dump in the orzo and cook for 6 minutes – you're not fully cooking it through just yet. Scoop out and retain about 3 tablespoons of the cooking water and then drain the semi-cooked pasta in a sieve and leave to one side until ready to use.

Lay the tomatoes on a baking tray, sprinkle with a little salt and pepper and cook under the hot grill for 5 minutes. Turn off the heat and leave the tomatoes to keep warm.

Melt the coconut oil in a large saucepan over a high heat. Add the leek, garlic and chicken and cook, stirring regularly, for 3 minutes. Squeeze in the tomato puree and continue frying, stirring regularly, for 1 minute, then pour in the chicken stock and bring up to the boil.

Now add your orzo to the pan with the chicken, along with the saved cooking water. Give the whole lot a stir, clamp on a lid, turn the heat down to medium and cook for 4 minutes.

Take the lid off and give the mix a stir – the pasta and chicken should both be cooked through by now. Check the chicken is cooked by slicing into one of the larger pieces to make sure the meat is white all the way through, with no raw pink bits left.

Stir in the chopped herbs and lemon juice along with a good pinch of salt and pepper.

Serve up your orzotto topped with the grilled tomatoes.

BAKED GNOCCHI WITH MINCED BEEF

SERVES 4

POST-WORKOUT

LONGER RECIPE

INGREDIENTS

1½ tbsp coconut oil
1kg lean beef mince
1 onion, diced
1 large carrot, diced
2 celery sticks, diced
2 sprigs of thyme
1 bay leaf
1 tbsp tomato puree
1 beef stock cube
salt and pepper
400g tinned chopped tomatoes
500g gnocchi
2 large handfuls of baby
  spinach leaves
green salad, to serve

A longer recipe (45 minutes) but perfect for a family of four. Kids and adults will love it. Don't be tempted to grate a load of cheese over this dish, though – it's a post-workout meal and we want to keep the fat content low.

METHOD

Melt half a tablespoon of the coconut oil in a large casserole dish or saucepan over a high heat. Crumble in half of the beef, brown it all over and then scrape it into a sieve over a bowl to drain off the excess fat. Repeat the process with a little more coconut oil and the rest of the beef.

Wipe the pan clean, add the remaining coconut oil and melt it over a medium to high heat. Add the onion, carrot and celery and fry, stirring regularly, for 3 minutes. Drop in the thyme and bay leaf and continue stir-frying for another minute before squeezing in the tomato puree and stirring it into the rest of the ingredients.

Tip the beef back into the pan and crumble in the stock cube along with some salt and pepper, the tomatoes and 100ml of water. Bring to the boil, then simmer for 15 minutes.

While the beef is simmering, bring a large saucepan of water to the boil and preheat your oven to 190°C (fan 170°C, gas mark 5). Once the water is boiling, tumble in the gnocchi and cook according to the packet instructions, then drain in a colander.

Tip the gnocchi straight into the pan with the simmering beef, turn off the heat and then stir through the spinach, leaving it to wilt in the residual heat.

Spoon everything into a large baking dish and bake in the oven for 20 minutes, or until the top sets a little and the edges start to crisp up.

Serve the gnocchi with a big bowl of salad.

SOUTHERN-STYLE QUINOA-COATED CHICKEN WITH WEDGES

SERVES 1

POST-WORKOUT
LONGER RECIPE

INGREDIENTS

1 sweet potato, peeled and
  sliced into 6 wedges
1 x 220g skinless chicken
  breast fillet
125g pre-cooked quinoa
2 tsp smoked paprika
1 tsp garlic granules
2 tsp onion granules
1 tsp dried oregano
1 egg
½ tbsp coconut oil
green salad, to serve
lemon wedges, to serve

If you're craving fried chicken and chips, quickly dive into
the kitchen and make this recipe instead. It tastes awesome and
won't make you feel guilteeee afterwards because it's so lean.
It takes longer than the usual 15 minutes (more like 25) but
I guarantee it is well worth the wait.

METHOD

Zap the sweet potato wedges in your microwave for 4 minutes,
rest for 2 minutes, then blast for another 4 minutes.

Meanwhile, place the chicken between two pieces of cling film or
baking parchment on a chopping board. Using a rolling pin, meat
mallet or any other blunt instrument, bash the chicken until it is
about 1cm thick all over.

Mix the quinoa, paprika, garlic granules, onion granules and
dried oregano together in a bowl and then tip the mixture onto
a plate, spreading it out a little.

Crack the egg into a separate bowl and whisk with a fork. Dip the
chicken into the egg, making sure as much of the flesh is covered
as possible. Lay the eggy chicken in the spiced quinoa mixture
and press it down to make sure the breast is coated all over.

Melt half of the coconut oil in one frying pan and the other half
in a second, both over a medium to high heat. Lay the chicken
down in one and the sweet potato wedges in the second. The
chicken will need about 4 minutes on each side, while the wedges
will be ready when they are browned all over. Check the chicken
is cooked by slicing into a thicker part to make sure the meat is
white all the way through, with no raw pink bits left.

When you're ready to eat, blot both the chicken and the wedges
with a piece of kitchen roll before serving. Dish up your fried
chicken and wedges with a side salad and lemon wedges.

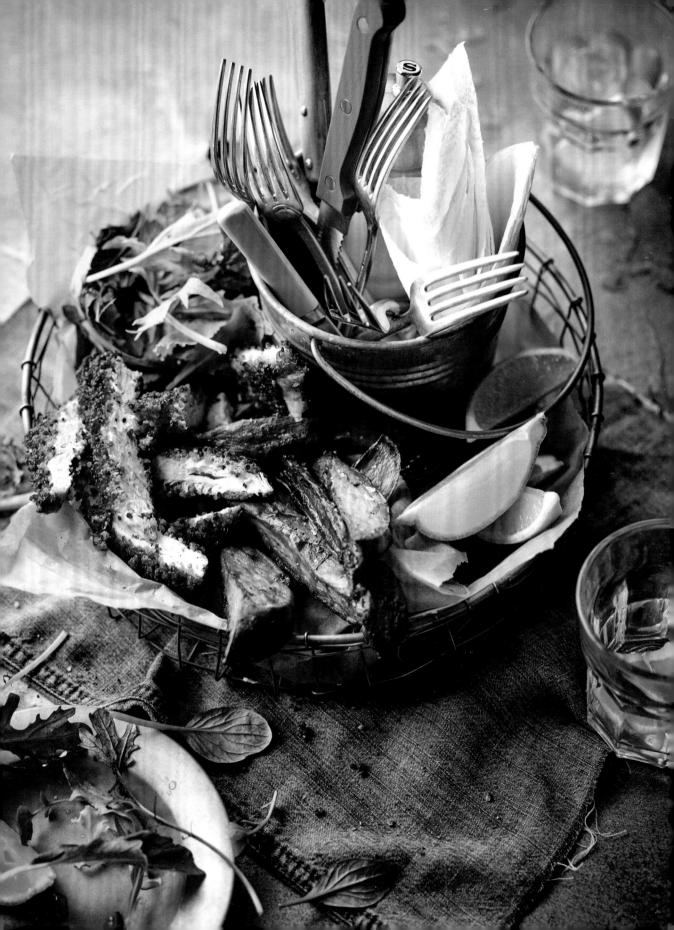

RICE AND CHICKEN STUFFED PEPPERS

POST-WORKOUT
LONGER RECIPE
INGREDIENTS

4 red peppers
½ tbsp coconut oil
2 celery sticks, diced
½ red onion, diced
1 carrot, diced
450g skinless chicken breast
   fillets, sliced into 1cm strips
2 tsp smoked paprika
2 tsp ground cumin
2 tsp celery salt
350g pre-cooked rice
100g tinned chickpeas, drained
   and rinsed
large handful of parsley,
   roughly chopped
green salad, to serve

An oldie, but a goldie. Instagram went gangbusters when
I first shared this recipe a year ago. I remember thinking,
right, that's a winner. I'll put that in Book 3. This one will take
you 40 minutes.

METHOD

Preheat your oven to 190°C (fan 170°C, gas mark 5).

Cut off the top and bottom of each pepper. Keep the tops, but
dice up the bases, which can be chucked into the rice mix later.
Use a sharp knife to remove the seeds and white parts from
inside the peppers – this should be really easy with the tops and
bottoms removed. Stand the peppers upright on a baking tray
and cook in the oven for 8 minutes, until just starting to soften.

While the peppers are cooking, melt the coconut oil in a large
frying pan over a high heat. Add the celery, onion and carrot
and stir-fry for 3 minutes. Slide in the chicken and continue to
stir-fry over the high heat for 2 minutes – try to get a bit of
colour on the chicken.

Don't forget to keep an eye on the peppers and take them out of
the oven when they're ready, but leave them on the baking tray.

Reduce the heat under the pan a little and sprinkle in the paprika,
cumin and celery salt, tossing everything together to season evenly.
Add the rice, crumbling it between your fingers as you drop it in,
and the chickpeas, quickly followed by 2 tablespoons of water.
Stir-fry for 2 minutes, or until the rice grains have separated. Take
the pan from the heat and stir through the parsley.

Fill the peppers with as much of the rice mixture as you can –
don't worry if some spills over the sides; it will go satisfyingly
crisp in the oven. When you've packed the peppers, slide them
back into the oven and bake for a further 10 minutes.

Serve up the stuffed peppers with a crisp green salad.

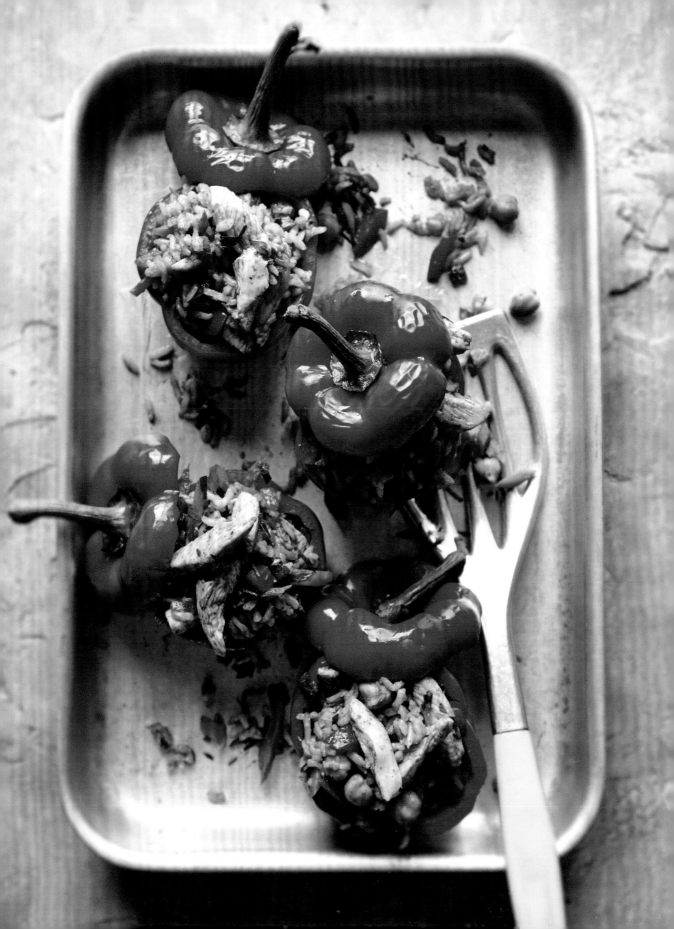

POST-WORKOUT
LONGER RECIPE
INGREDIENTS

1 tbsp coconut oil

2 large potatoes, each sliced
  into 6 wedges

salt and pepper

50g flour

2 eggs

150g fresh breadcrumbs

2 x 240g skinless cod fillets

125g frozen peas

5 mint leaves

1 lemon

1 red chilli, de-seeded and
  finely sliced

green salad, to serve

FISH AND CHIPS WITH MUSHY PEAS

Another firm takeaway favourite, but I've given it the Body Coach makeover to keep it lean and healthy. Rather than go to the greasy fish and chip shop this week, try this instead. It will take you 45 minutes.

METHOD

Preheat your oven to 190°C (fan 170°C, gas mark 5).

Dollop the coconut oil onto a baking tray and slide it into the oven to melt. Carefully lay the potato wedges in the hot oil, season with salt and pepper and roast in the oven for 20 minutes, turning halfway through.

While the potatoes are roasting, tip the flour into a bowl and mix in a generous amount of salt and pepper. Crack the eggs into a separate bowl and beat them well with a fork. Tip the breadcrumbs into another bowl.

Dab the first fish fillet into the flour – you want to give it a decent coating, but with no clumps, so dust and pat to remove the excess. Next dip the fish into the beaten egg, again making sure you get decent coverage. Then drop the fish into the breadcrumbs, pressing down to make sure the crumbs stick. Dip the fish back into the egg and then back into the crumbs to give it a double crumb layer. Repeat the process with the second fillet.

When the potatoes have had their 20-minute head start, remove the tray from the oven and make room to gently slide on the crumbed fish. Roast them together for a further 20 minutes, turning both the fish and the potatoes once during that time.

While the fish and chips are baking, boil the peas together with the mint leaves in a pan of water for 3 minutes. Before draining, scoop out about 50ml of the cooking liquid and keep to one side. Drain the peas and mint in a sieve or colander, then tip them back into the pan. Add the juice of half the lemon, the chilli, a decent pinch of salt and pepper and the reserved cooking liquid. Roughly mash up the minty peas with a potato masher.

Serve up the fish, chips and mushy peas with wedges of lemon and a green salad.

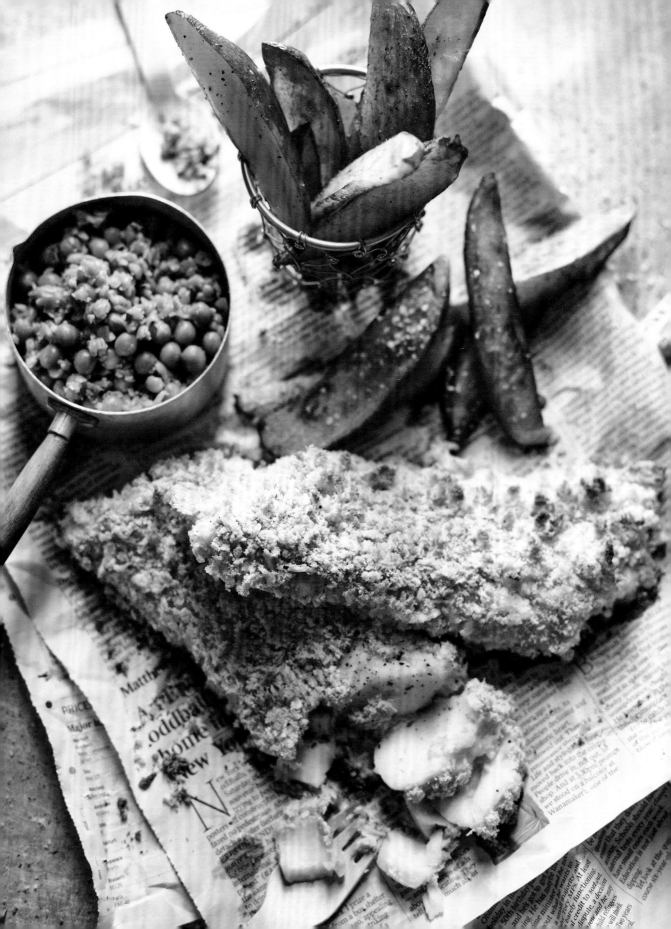

SNACKS AND TREATS

5

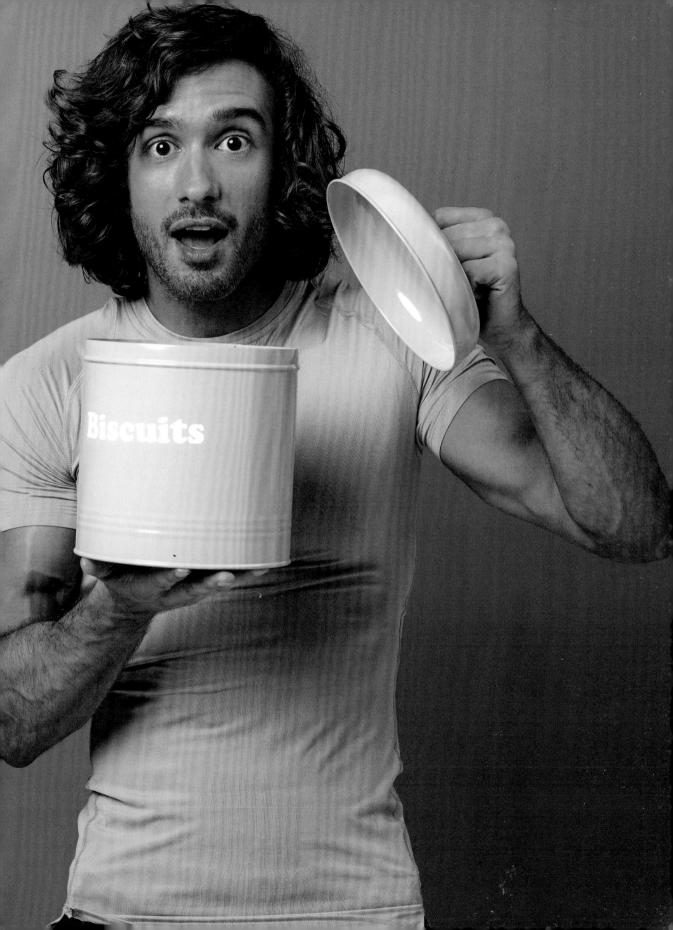

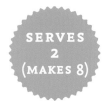

MAKE AHEAD
GOOD TO FREEZE
INGREDIENTS

1 carrot, grated
75g cooked quinoa
1 egg
30g flour
½ tsp ground cumin
½ tbsp coconut oil
2 tbsp light soy sauce
1 tbsp rice wine vinegar

QUINOA AND CARROT FRITTERS

Ready in minutes, devoured in seconds. These are a great little snack to stop the mid-morning hunger pangs and keep you going until lunch.

METHOD

Mix together the carrot, quinoa, egg, flour and cumin in a bowl with 1 tablespoon of water until it all becomes a big orange mush.

Melt a little of the coconut oil in a non-stick frying pan over a medium to high heat. Dollop in the carrot mixture in mounds of 2 tablespoons and flatten them out with the back of your spoon. I normally manage to fit three in my pan at the same time; sometimes I'll squeeze in four, then sometimes I just make two massive ones!

Fry the fritters for 3 minutes on each side, or until they are cooked through and golden brown. Repeat the process with the rest of the oil and batter.

Just before serving, mix together the soy sauce and vinegar for a perfectly zingy dip.

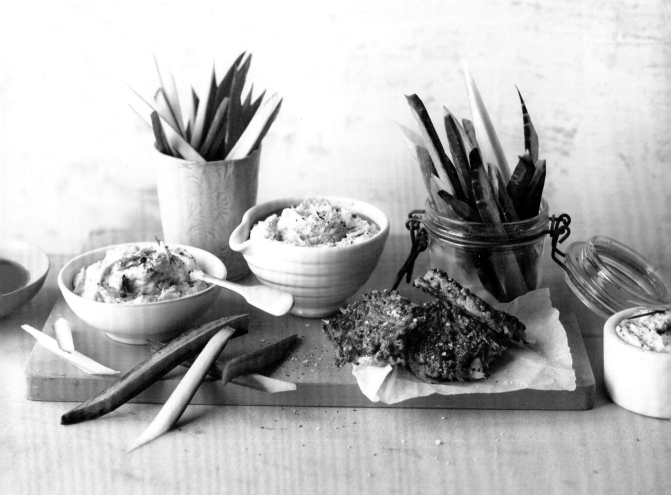

ROASTED CAULIFLOWER HUMMUS

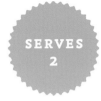

SERVES 2

MAKE AHEAD
LONGER RECIPE
INGREDIENTS

½ head of cauliflower,
   florets only
2 tbsp olive oil
salt
2 cloves garlic, peeled
juice of 2 lemons
1 x 400g tin of chickpeas,
   drained (roughly 240g)
2 tbsp unsweetened peanut
   butter
½ tsp ground cumin
raw vegetable batons, to serve

Something quite magical happens to cauliflower when it is roasted. It takes on a new persona and tastes so much better than normal. This is a great mid-afternoon snack which takes 45 minutes to make and will keep in the fridge for up to 4 days, no problem.

METHOD

Preheat your oven to 190°C (fan 170°C, gas mark 5).

Dump the cauliflower florets into a roasting tray, drizzle with the olive oil and season with salt. Roast the cauliflower for 10 minutes on its own and then add the garlic and roast for a further 10 minutes.

When roasted, carefully spoon the florets and garlic into a blender and add the lemon juice, chickpeas, peanut butter, cumin and about 75ml of warm water. Blitz until smooth.

Serve the dip straight away with raw vegetable batons (see picture on previous page), or leave to cool and store in an airtight container in the fridge.

SERVES
1

MAKE AHEAD
INGREDIENTS

1 tsp butter
3 spring onions, finely sliced
1 clove garlic, finely chopped
250g chestnut mushrooms,
  roughly chopped into small
  pieces
salt and pepper
60g ground almonds
50g cream cheese
juice of 1 lemon
large handful of chives, finely
  sliced
raw vegetable batons, to serve

SERVES
2

MAKE AHEAD
INGREDIENTS

1 ripe avocado, roughly
  chopped
125g smoked salmon, roughly
  chopped
35g crème fraiche
2 tsp sesame seed oil
juice of 1 lemon
handful of chives, finely
  chopped
raw vegetables, to serve

GARLIC MUSHROOM AND ALMOND DIP

This may seem like an odd combination, but give it a try because it tastes great and contains good fats. It will keep in the fridge for up to 3 days in an airtight container.

METHOD

Melt the butter in a large frying pan over a high heat. Add the spring onions, garlic and mushrooms and fry for 2 minutes, stirring almost constantly.

Season with salt and pepper and cover the pan with a lid (if you don't have one big enough then just use a plate) and reduce the heat a little. Leave the ingredients to cook in their own juices for 5 minutes, by which time they should be soft.

Tip the mushroom mixture into a food processor and blitz until roughly smooth – it's nice to have a bit of texture. Tip into a bowl, add all the remaining ingredients apart from the vegetable batons and mix everything together.

It's ready to eat now (see picture on previous page) or alternatively, leave it to cool completely, refrigerate and save for later.

CHEAT'S TARAMASALATA

Taramasalata is normally made with smoked fish roe, but I like to use smoked salmon instead. Weird as it may sound, I love dunking raw cauliflower into this dip.

METHOD

Place all the ingredients, apart from the raw vegetables, into a food processor and blitz until roughly smooth.

Tip the dip into a bowl and serve up with chopped raw veggies (see picture on previous page).

CHOCOLATE PROTEIN CREPES WITH STRAWBERRY SAUCE

SERVES
2
(MAKES 8)

These need very little introduction. If like me you've got a sweet tooth and get cravings, then these are just what you need.

INGREDIENTS

125g strawberries, quartered
1 tbsp runny honey
110g plain flour
2 scoops (60g) chocolate protein powder
2 eggs
325ml almond milk
1 tbsp coconut oil
a little cocoa powder, for dusting – optional

METHOD

Drop the strawberries into a small saucepan and squeeze in the honey. Put the pan on a medium heat and cook for about 10 minutes, or until the strawberries take on a sauce-like consistency.

While the strawberries are simmering away, place the flour, protein powder, eggs and almond milk into a food processor and blitz until smooth.

Melt a little of the coconut oil (1 tablespoon should be more than enough for all the pancakes) in a medium non-stick frying pan over a high heat. Pour in a ladleful of the batter and immediately pick up the pan and swirl the mix to coat the base of the frying pan.

Fry the crepe for about 1 minute before flipping and frying for 1 minute on the other side. Don't worry – the first one is always the worst!

Repeat the process with the remaining coconut oil and batter. I like to fold my crepes into triangles and pile them up to be topped with a dusting of cocoa powder and the warm strawberry sauce.

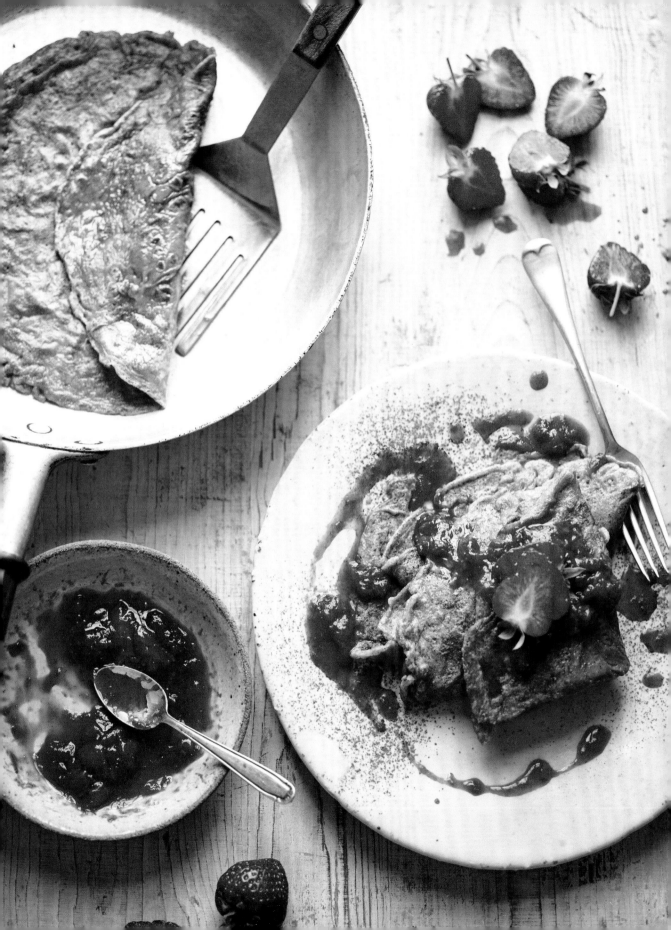

JOE'S PEANUT BUTTER BROWNIES

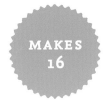

MAKES 16

MAKE AHEAD
LONGER RECIPE

INGREDIENTS

140g dark chocolate (over 70 per cent cocoa), broken into small pieces
60g unsweetened peanut butter
20g honey
2 over-ripe bananas, peeled and roughly chopped
2 scoops (60g) chocolate protein powder
30ml almond milk
splash of vanilla extract
3 eggs, yolks separated
cocoa powder for dusting – optional

These brownies are a really naughty treat which will make you want to shout 'Guilteeee!' when you try them for the first time. Be sure to use chocolate with a high cocoa content. It may seem weird, but over-ripe bananas that are brown on the outside will work best. This recipe will take 25 minutes.

METHOD

Put the kettle on to boil. Preheat your oven to 160°C (fan 140°C, gas mark 3) and line an 18cm brownie tray with baking parchment.

Put the chocolate in a large bowl along with the peanut butter and honey. Sit the bowl on top of a saucepan of boiling water and melt. Don't let the base of the bowl touch the simmering water.

Meanwhile, blitz the bananas in a blender until almost smooth, then scrape into a clean bowl. Add the protein powder, almond milk, vanilla extract and egg yolks and mix together.

When the chocolate and peanut butter have melted, remove the bowl from the heat and stir in the banana mixture.

Next, whisk the egg whites until they are stiff. Stir a third into the chocolate batter and then, using a gentle chopping action, fold in the rest of the egg whites.

Spoon the batter into the brownie tray and bake in the oven for 12 minutes.

Remove from the oven and leave to cool for 5 minutes before chunking up into 16 large squares and dusting with cocoa powder, if using.

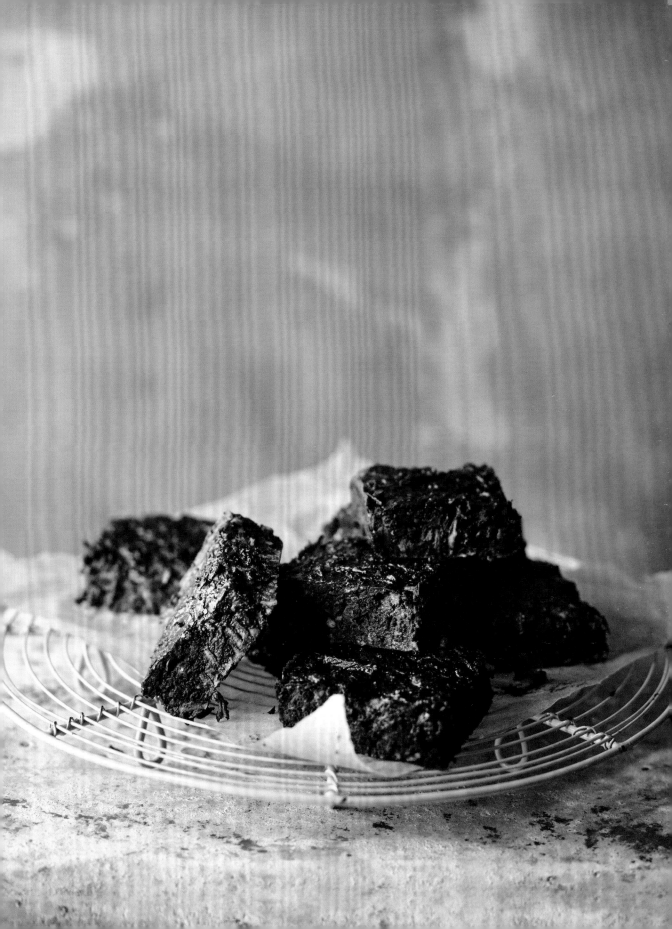

MAKE AHEAD
LONGER RECIPE
(quick to make but needs to
set overnight in the freezer)

INGREDIENTS

1 banana, chopped into 2cm
   chunks
200g frozen berries (I like a
   summer berry mix)
1 tbsp almond butter
200g reduced-fat Greek
   yoghurt
drizzle of honey, to serve

FROZEN BERRY YOGHURT

Frozen yoghurt tastes good any time of the year, so why not treat yourself to this one at home? I like to keep a box of chopped bananas in the freezer so that I can make this in minutes.

METHOD

Spread the banana chunks out on a tray lined with baking parchment and put into the freezer to freeze solid overnight.

When you're ready to make and eat your treat, place the frozen banana into a blender with all the remaining ingredients except the honey and blitz until they reach the consistency of frozen yoghurt.

Serve with a drizzle of honey.

CHOCOLATE AND PROTEIN MOUSSE

INGREDIENTS

175ml water
200g dark chocolate
  (minimum 70% cocoa),
  broken into small pieces
2 scoops (60g) chocolate or
  vanilla protein powder
a tray of ice

This is the recipe to break out when you fancy a nice choccy treat. It's a rich chocolate mousse that contains only chocolate, water and protein powder, so it's super-easy to make and tastes lovely.

METHOD

Bring the water to the boil in a saucepan.

You will need two bowls: one medium-sized into which you'll place the chocolate and protein powder; and a second slightly larger one into which the first bowl will fit comfortably.

Tip the ice into the larger bowl and pour in enough cold water to just cover the ice.

When the water has boiled, pour half of it into the chocolate and protein powder bowl and whisk together until the chocolate has melted. Pour in the remaining water and stir.

Next, carefully lower the chocolate-filled bowl into the larger bowl with the ice and start whisking the chocolate again.

As it cools, the chocolate will become thicker and thicker until it resembles a mousse. Scoop this straight out into a bowl and start eating.

The mousse will begin to collapse after about 10 minutes, but I don't think it will last that long!

MAKE AHEAD
LONGER RECIPE

INGREDIENTS

1 tsp coconut oil
120g porridge oats
180g raspberries
4 eggs
200ml reduced-fat Greek yoghurt
1 scoop (30g) vanilla protein powder
2 tbsp honey
½ tsp baking powder
45g plain flour

RASPBERRY CLAFOUTIS

There are not many puddings better than a clafoutis and I thought I would try to make a healthier, less fiddly version. It should take you 20 minutes and, like all tasty things, it does contain quite a lot of sugar, so eat this as a treat every now and again and be sure to share it.

METHOD

Preheat your oven to 190°C (fan 170°C, gas mark 5).

Grease a small ovenproof dish with the coconut oil and then sprinkle over half of the porridge oats, making sure some of them stick to the sides as well as the base. Tumble the raspberries in an even layer over the top.

Whisk together the remaining ingredients and carefully pour over the raspberries. Scatter over the remaining oats and bake for 20 minutes until brown and set.

Serve up while warm, or leave to cool for later.

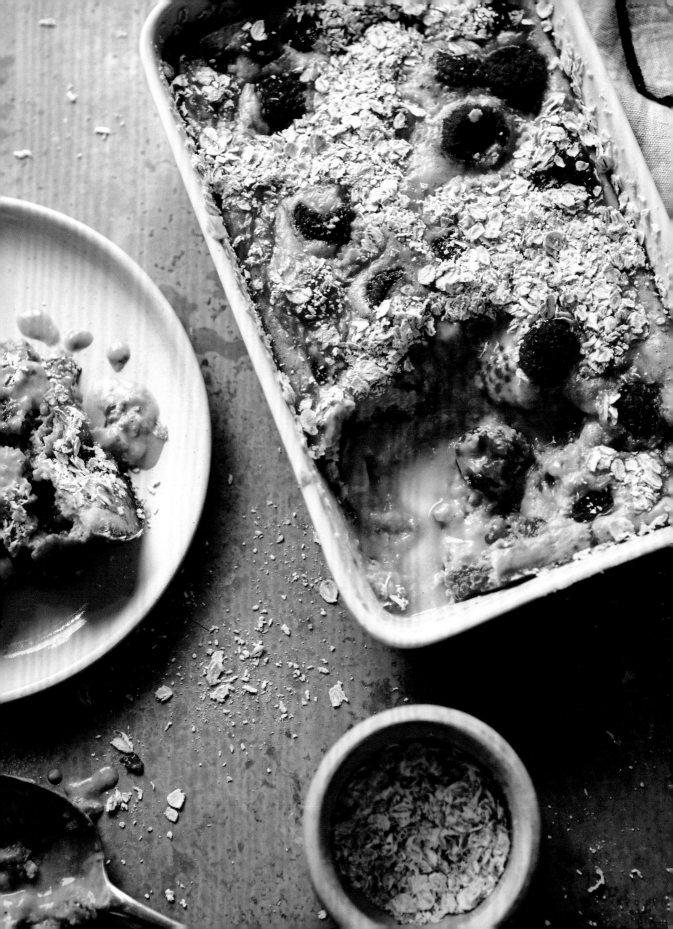

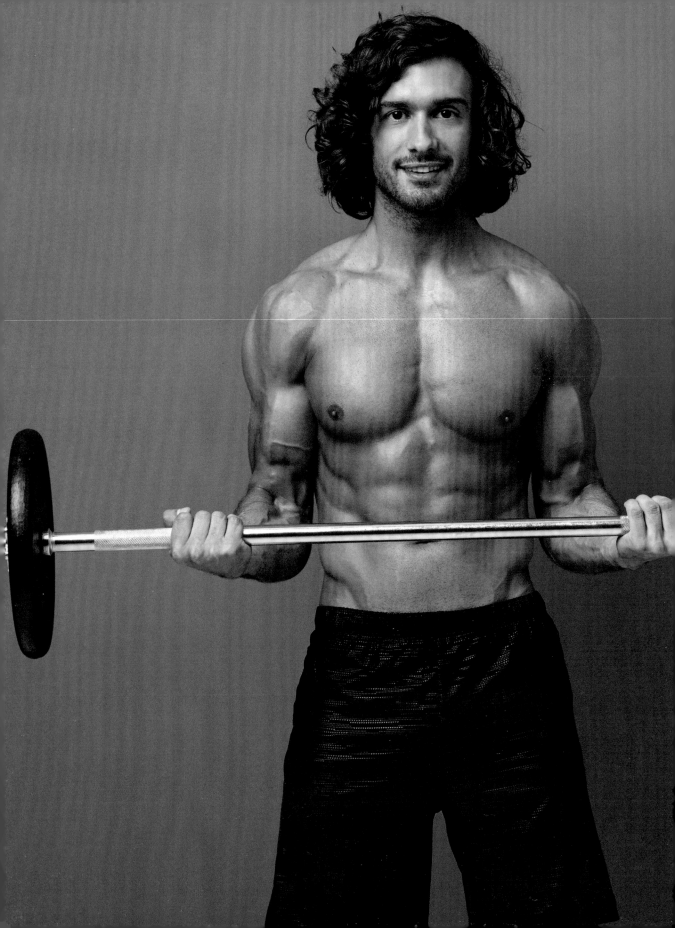

6

PYRAMID
RESISTANCE
HIIT
TRAINING

BUILDING MUSCLE AND BURNING FAT

///

I hope you're ready to feel the burn because these workouts are intense! It's going to be tough and sweaty and you'll probably be cursing my name during the final sets, but trust me, it's worth the effort when you see the effect it will have on your physique. This is one of my favourite training cycles from the 90 Day Shift, Shape and Sustain Plan because it builds both lean muscle and strength. And when you combine these high-volume resistance sessions with HIIT cardio, it will have your body melting fat for fun so you can stay lean all year round.

That's what you want, right? No more up-and-down battles with your weight, or panicking four weeks before your holiday. I want you to get lean, strong, confident and happy and maintain that feeling for the long term. It is possible, and you can and will achieve it if you commit and dedicate yourself to the Lean in 15 lifestyle and boss this training plan.

In Book 1, *The Shift Plan*, we focused on burning fat and improving fitness with HIIT cardio. Then in Book 2, *The Shape Plan*, we progressed by combining German Volume Training (GVT) with HIIT to build lean muscle and shape your physique. This involved performing 10 sets of 10 reps per muscle group, which was a challenge in itself. Now let me introduce you to phase three – Pyramid Resistance HIIT – where we step it up another gear. You'll be performing up to 300 reps per session, with a combination of low reps and high reps to really shock your muscles. This volume of training will force your muscle fibres to break down and, when they repair, they will grow back bigger and stronger, leaving you with a leaner physique.

Remember, your target should always be to build and maintain as much lean muscle as possible because lean muscle tissue is more metabolically active than body fat. This means that the leaner you are, the greater your resting metabolic rate will be. Which results in your body burning more calories at rest and therefore means you can enjoy more food and sustain your progress.

Please note that due to their volume and intensity, these workouts are not for complete beginners. If you do attempt to go all Arnie and bust out 300 squats in one session, trust me, you'll be in a world of pain. You'll be walking like John Wayne for about a week, so please take my advice and gradually build up your strength with body-weight exercises before starting this training plan. If you're a complete beginner, you can check out my YouTube channel for beginners' HIIT workouts. Once you've reached a good level of fitness, you can then start incorporating weight training into your routine and build up your strength. Then, once you've got some iron mileage under your belt, you can step up to these pyramid resistance sessions safely and with confidence.

Even if you can't do the pyramid training right now, you can still enjoy the recipes in this book as long as you're doing some form of training, whether it's HIIT or GVT.

WHAT IS HIIT CARDIO?

Just in case you're not sure what HIIT cardio is, I'll quickly give you the lowdown. It's grown in popularity over the past few years and suddenly everyone seems to be doing it. I'm a big fan. It's hard work but it keeps me lean and makes me feel great afterwards. HIIT stands for high intensity interval training and it involves short bursts of maximum effort followed by a less intense rest or recovery period. For example, 30 seconds of all-out sprinting followed by a 45-second walk or complete rest. You then repeat this for about 15–20 minutes. It doesn't seem like much but it's extremely effective at burning fat because, unlike low intensity steady-state cardio such as jogging, it creates an intense after-burn which means your body uses up calories for hours after you've completed the workout. This can help your body create an energy deficit in half the time, which makes it perfect for busy people. Also, because it's so taxing on your cardiovascular system, it gets you super-fit really fast. Always check with your doctor before starting a new exercise regime if you have any health concerns.

> ❝ONCE YOU'VE REACHED A GOOD LEVEL OF FITNESS, YOU CAN START INCORPORATING WEIGHT TRAINING❞

HIIT should never be easy and, remember, the more intense the workout, the greater the after-burn effect, so really push hard in those 30-second working sets.

The principles of HIIT can be applied to any cardio machine, such as a treadmill, cross-trainer, rower or exercise bike. Or to any body-weight exercises, such as burpees, mountain climbers, hill sprints and skipping.

WHAT EQUIPMENT WILL I NEED?

If you're not a member of a gym, to complete the four workouts in this book you will need to invest in an exercise bench and a set of adjustable dumbbells or barbells. This is because you will be increasing and reducing the weights you lift as you go through the various rep ranges.

HOW OFTEN WILL I TRAIN?

You will aim to do four workouts per week and take three full rest days. Trust me, you'll need these rest days to recover and repair your muscles. The good news is you will still be burning fat on rest days, so enjoy them!

Aim to complete all four sessions each week to ensure you get a full-body workout. Avoid trying to be a hero by doing more than one workout per day. One of these sessions is more than enough. I also advise not training more than two days in a row. The rest and recovery days are just as important, if not more so, than the workout days, so please don't skip them.

In my opinion, the best weekly format would be:

MONDAY	TUESDAY	WEDNESDAY	THURSDAY	FRIDAY	SATURDAY	SUNDAY
Chest and back	Arms	Rest	Legs	Rest	Shoulders and abs	Rest

WARM UP

It's really important not to miss your warm-up: it ensures your muscles and joints are properly prepared and helps to avoid injuries. Before you begin your HIIT, carry out an exercise-specific warm-up. If, for example, you are starting with treadmill sprints, then spend a couple of minutes power walking. Make the most of your training and warm up!

HOW DO I DO IT?

You are going to combine two rounds of weight training with two rounds of HIIT cardio intervals per session. First, complete a round of pyramid resistance training, rest for 2–3 minutes and then go straight into a round of HIIT. Then repeat. One HIIT round will consist of four 30-second maximum effort intervals, with a 45-second rest interval between each effort.

The first round of weight training will be an ascending pyramid. This means that as the number of repetitions decreases, the weight you lift will increase.

For example:

Reps	Weight
50	30kg
40	35kg
30	40kg
20	45kg
10	50kg

The weights here are for an experienced trainer – I would recommend starting with a weight you're comfortable with and increasing it bit by bit. Don't be discouraged if you have to kick off with 5kg and work up.

The second round of weight training will be a descending pyramid: as the number of repetitions increases, you will reduce the weight you lift.

For example:

Reps	Weight
10	50kg
20	45kg
30	40kg
40	35kg
50	30kg

GO AND GET LEAN

Good luck with your training. The workouts will be intense, so dig deep on both the HIIT section and the weight training. Your body will not change unless you give it a good reason to, so go and attack every session with 100 per cent effort. Consistency is key – don't be disheartened if you don't see results right away. Think long term with this plan and keep going.

PICK YOUR HIIT

Choose from any of the following 4 exercises to build into your session

///////////////////////////

HIIT option
1. Burpees

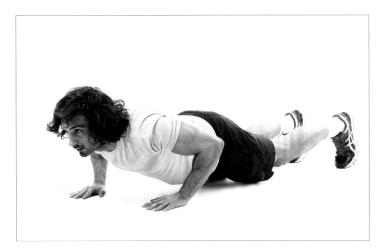

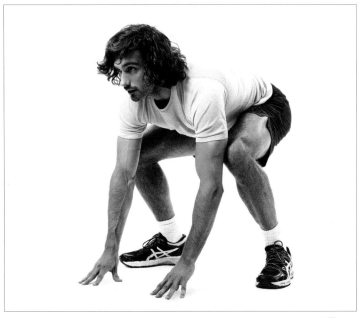

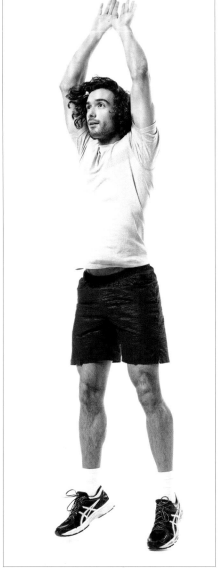

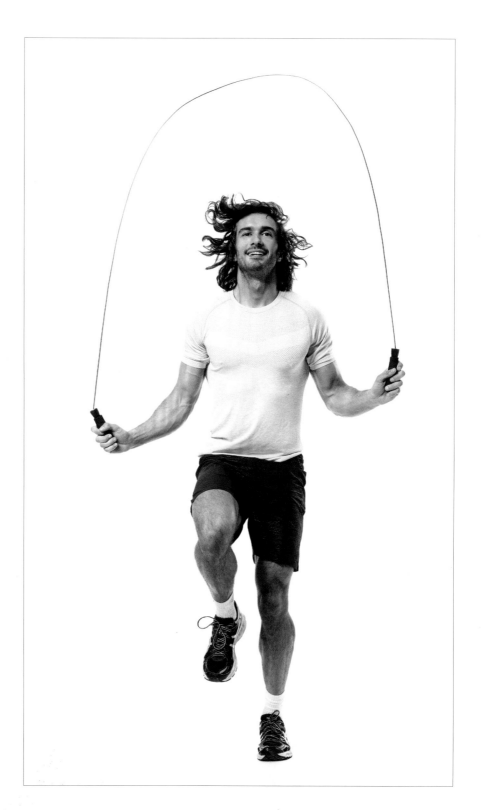

3. Running on the spot with punches

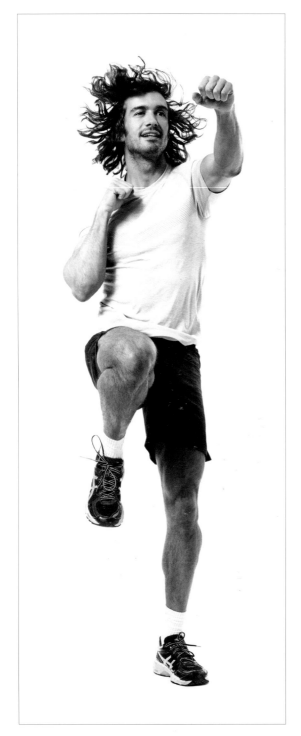
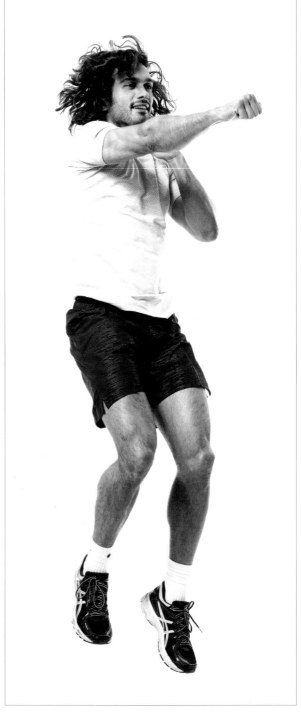

4. Mountain climbers

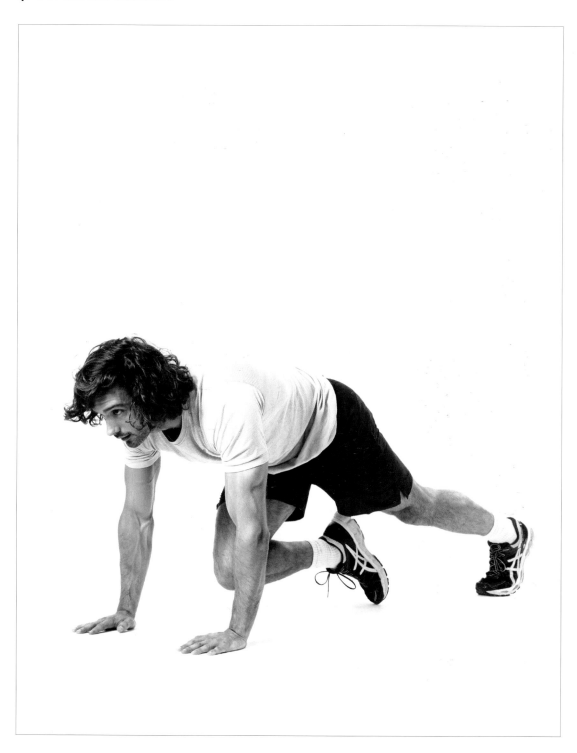

OPTION 1 – ARMS (BICEPS AND TRICEPS)

TRAINING DESCRIPTION	GUIDELINES
ROUND 1 Biceps **50 REPS – 30 SECS REST** **40 REPS – 45 SECS REST** **30 REPS – 60 SECS REST** **20 REPS – 90 SECS REST** **10 REPS – Round complete!**	Barbell curls
HIIT ROUND 1 (One working set followed by one resting set)	**WORKING SETS:** 4 **DURATION:** 30 SECS **MAX** (HEART RATE or EFFORT) **RESTING SETS:** 4 **DURATION:** 45 SECS Depending on your fitness levels this will either be a complete stop or around 25 per cent of your max effort.
ROUND 2 Triceps **10 REPS – 90 SECS REST** **20 REPS – 60 SECS REST** **30 REPS – 45 SECS REST** **40 REPS – 30 SECS REST** **50 REPS – Round complete!**	Lying tricep extensions
HIIT ROUND 2 (One working set followed by one resting set)	**WORKING SETS:** 4 **DURATION:** 30 SECS **MAX** (HEART RATE or EFFORT) **RESTING SETS:** 4 **DURATION:** 45 SECS Depending on your fitness levels this will either be a complete stop or around 25 per cent of your max effort.

Barbell curls

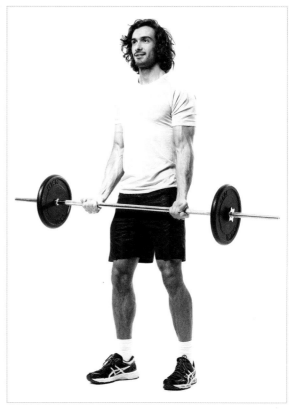

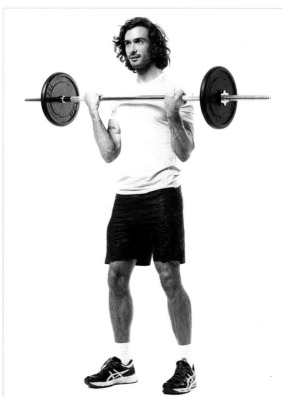

Lying tricep extensions

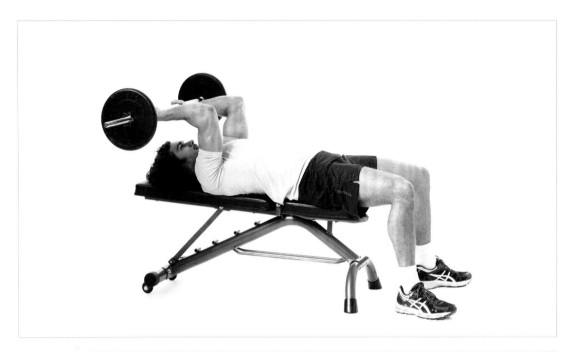

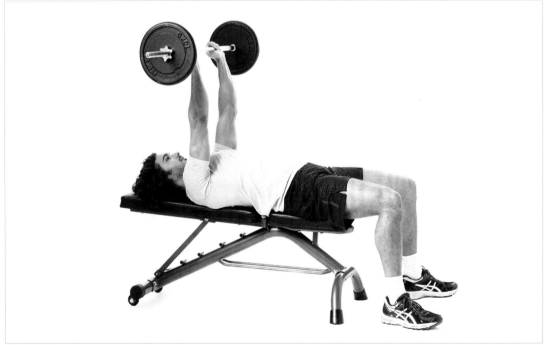

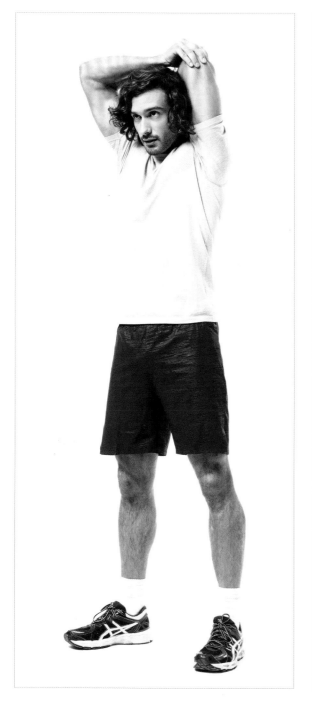

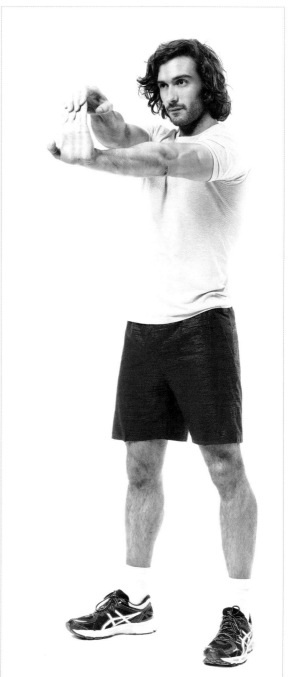

OPTION 2 – CHEST AND BACK

TRAINING DESCRIPTION	GUIDELINES
ROUND 1 Chest **50 REPS – 30 SECS REST** **40 REPS – 45 SECS REST** **30 REPS – 60 SECS REST** **20 REPS – 90 SECS REST** **10 REPS – Round complete!**	Incline dumbbell bench press
HIIT ROUND 1 (One working set followed by one resting set)	**WORKING SETS:** 4 **DURATION:** 30 SECS MAX (HEART RATE or EFFORT) **RESTING SETS:** 4 **DURATION:** 45 SECS Depending on your fitness levels this will either be a complete stop or around 25 per cent of your max effort.
ROUND 2 Back **10 REPS – 90 SECS REST** **20 REPS – 60 SECS REST** **30 REPS – 45 SECS REST** **40 REPS – 30 SECS REST** **50 REPS – Round complete!**	Bent-over dumbbell rows
HIIT ROUND 2 (One working set followed by one resting set)	**WORKING SETS:** 4 **DURATION:** 30 SECS MAX (HEART RATE or EFFORT) **RESTING SETS:** 4 **DURATION:** 45 SECS Depending on your fitness levels this will either be a complete stop or around 25 per cent of your max effort.

Incline dumbbell bench press

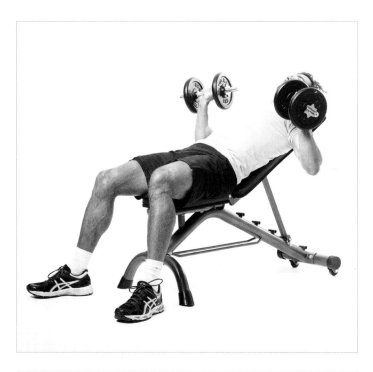

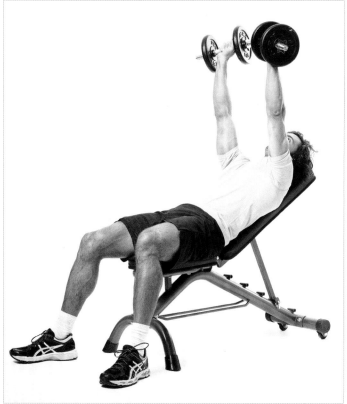

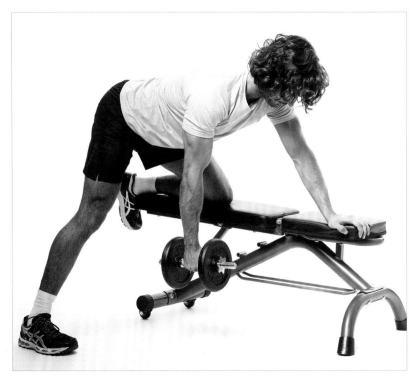

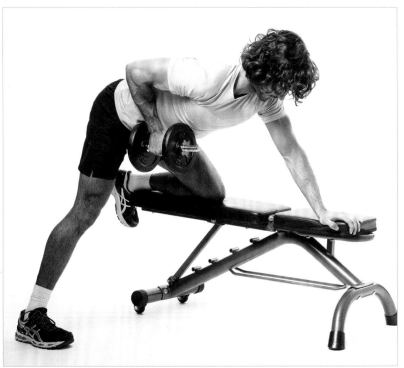

Cool-down stretch

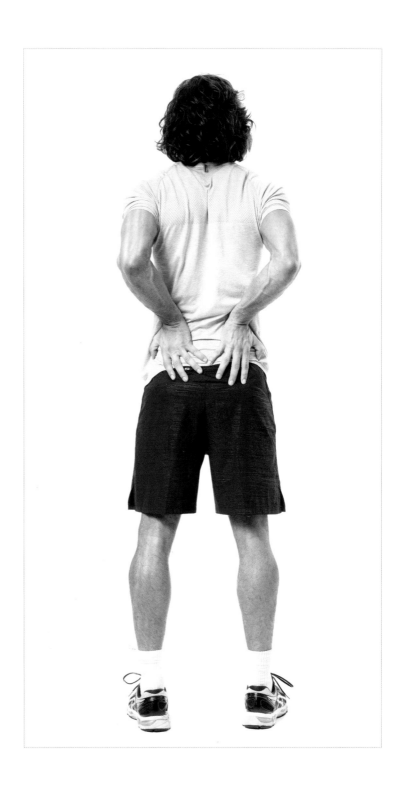

OPTION 3 – LEGS

TRAINING DESCRIPTION	GUIDELINES
ROUND 1 Legs **50 REPS – 30 SECS REST** **40 REPS – 45 SECS REST** **30 REPS – 60 SECS REST** **20 REPS – 90 SECS REST** **10 REPS – Round complete!**	Barbell front squats
HIIT ROUND 1 (One working set followed by one resting set)	**WORKING SETS:** 4 **DURATION:** 30 SECS MAX (HEART RATE or EFFORT) **RESTING SETS:** 4 **DURATION:** 45 SECS Depending on your fitness levels this will either be a complete stop or around 25 per cent of your max effort.
ROUND 2 Legs **10 REPS – 90 SECS REST** **20 REPS – 60 SECS REST** **30 REPS – 45 SECS REST** **40 REPS – 30 SECS REST** **50 REPS – Round complete!**	Barbell lunges
HIIT ROUND 2 (One working set followed by one resting set)	**WORKING SETS:** 4 **DURATION:** 30 SECS MAX (HEART RATE or EFFORT) **RESTING SETS:** 4 **DURATION:** 45 SECS Depending on your fitness levels this will either be a complete stop or around 25 per cent of your max effort.

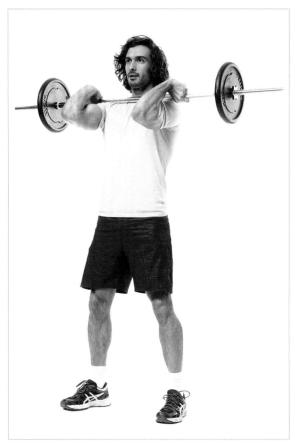

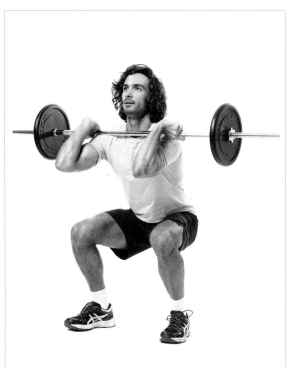

Barbell lunges

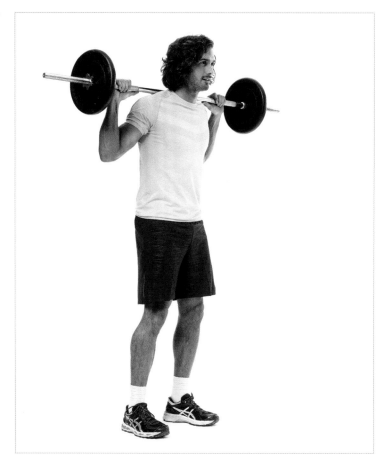

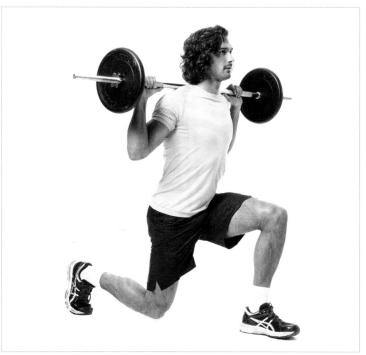

Cool-down stretch

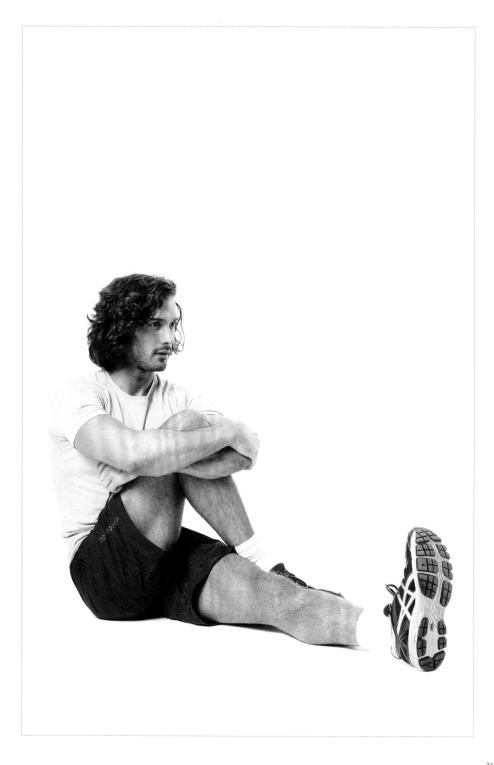

OPTION 4 – SHOULDERS AND ABS

TRAINING DESCRIPTION	GUIDELINES
ROUND 1 Shoulders **50 REPS – 30 SECS REST** **40 REPS – 45 SECS REST** **30 REPS – 60 SECS REST** **20 REPS – 90 SECS REST** **10 REPS – Round complete!**	Dumbbell shoulder press
HIIT ROUND 1 (One working set followed by one resting set)	**WORKING SETS:** 4 **DURATION:** 30 SECS **MAX (HEART RATE or EFFORT)** **RESTING SETS:** 4 **DURATION:** 45 SECS Depending on your fitness levels this will either be a complete stop or around 25 per cent of your max effort.
ROUND 2 Abs **10 REPS – 90 SECS REST** **20 REPS – 60 SECS REST** **30 REPS – 45 SECS REST** **40 REPS – 30 SECS REST** **50 REPS – Round complete!**	Bicycle crunches or Simple crunches
HIIT ROUND 2 (One working set followed by one resting set)	**WORKING SETS:** 4 **DURATION:** 30 SECS **MAX (HEART RATE or EFFORT)** **RESTING SETS:** 4 **DURATION:** 45 SECS Depending on your fitness levels this will either be a complete stop or around 25 per cent of your max effort.

Dumbbell shoulder press

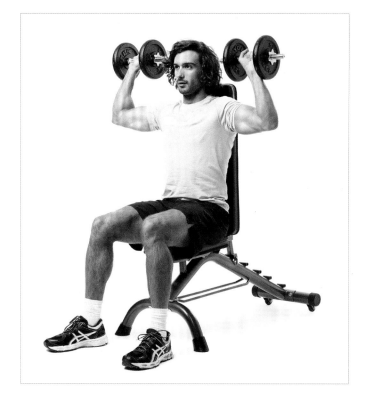

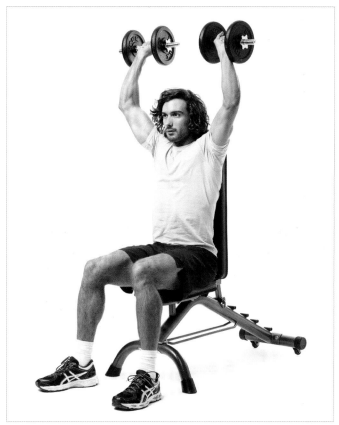

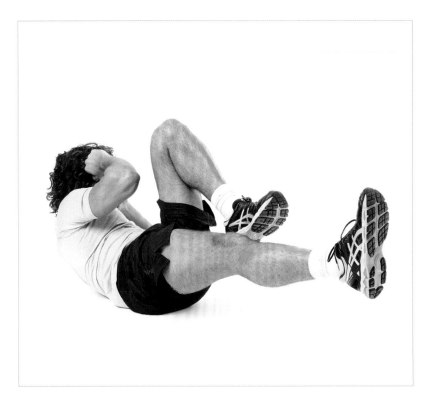

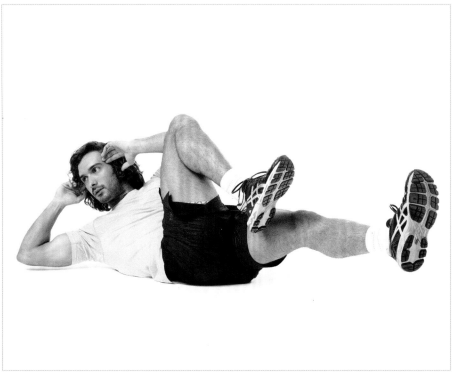

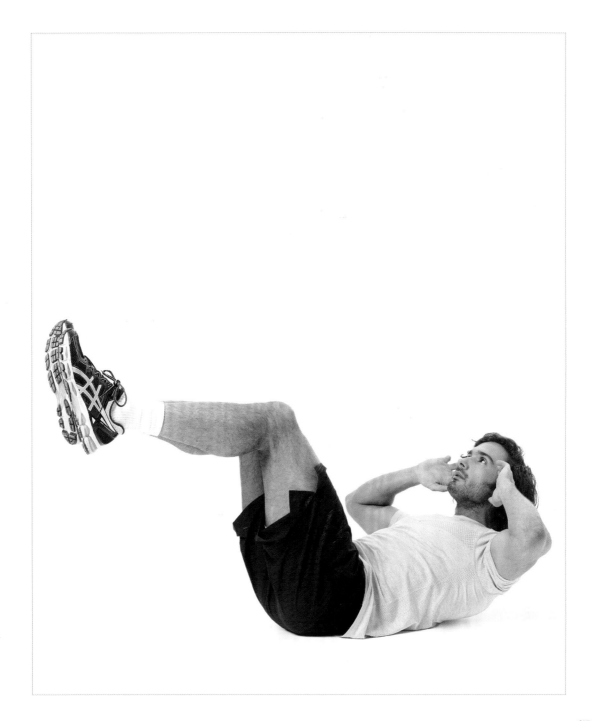

COOL DOWN
AND RECOVERY

//

As you can see, you will be completing 300 repetitions per
session, as well as a total of eight 30-second HIIT intervals.
This means your muscles are going to be getting really worked
over. When you lift weights you are effectively contracting
and shortening the muscles, and this makes stretching
post-workout essential for maintaining good flexibility and
mobility. My advice is to stretch out the muscle group you work
for at least 10 minutes after each session. Keep the stretches
specific to your workout. For example, if you do squats and
lunges, be sure to stretch your quads, glutes and hamstrings.
I know it's boring but it really is going to ease muscle soreness
and help with recovery, as well as reduce your risk of injury.

JOE'S POST-WORKOUT
PROTEIN SHAKE

As you can see on page 22, I always have a protein shake with
honey immediately after I train – it's great for muscle repair.

REDUCED-CARB

INGREDIENTS

1 scoop (30g) vanilla
  protein powder
15g honey
100g baby spinach leaves
handful of ice cubes

METHOD

Throw everything into a blender with a good splash of water
and blitz until smooth.

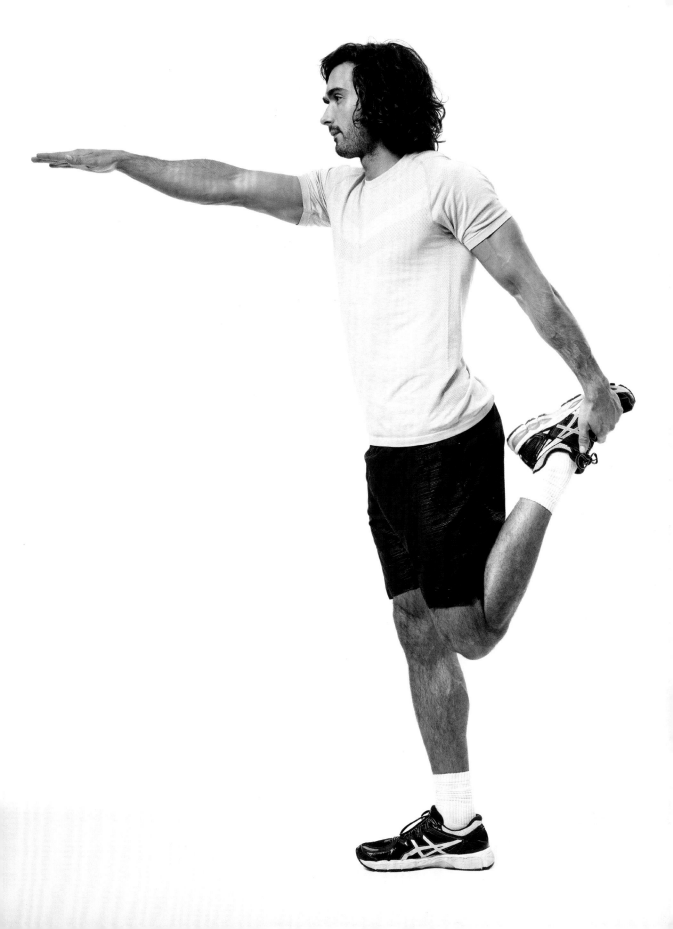

MY LEAN
WINNERS

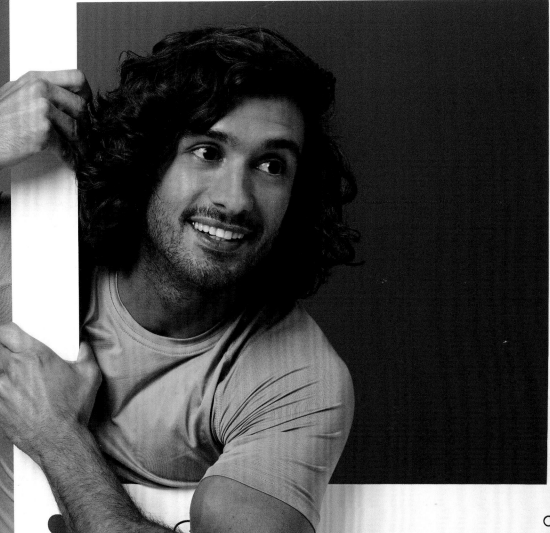

MY LEAN WINNERS

///

One of the highlights of my day is receiving new transformation pictures and testimonials from clients on my 90 Day Shift, Shape and Sustain Plan. This is when I get to see and read about the real impact my training plans and recipes are having on people's lives all over the world. Nothing makes me happier than knowing I've helped improve someone's health, fitness and self-confidence. I truly believe exercise and good nutrition is the key to feeling energized, positive and happy every day, and I'm really proud that my plan is giving this to people.

I've heard from people who've had difficulty conceiving but who followed the plan, lost weight and now send me pictures of them and their babies. Others have tackled eating disorders, IBS and type 2 diabetes. Many people have simply struggled for years on every single diet known to man, and after 90 days on my plan have transformed their body.

I've decided to include a few inspiring transformations from clients on my 90 Day Shift, Shape and Sustain Plan, which uses the same principles as in my books, but they follow a programme tailored to their individual energy needs. This takes into account factors such as their age, body composition, activity levels and past dieting history.

If you want to see more, visit my transformations gallery at thebodycoach.com.

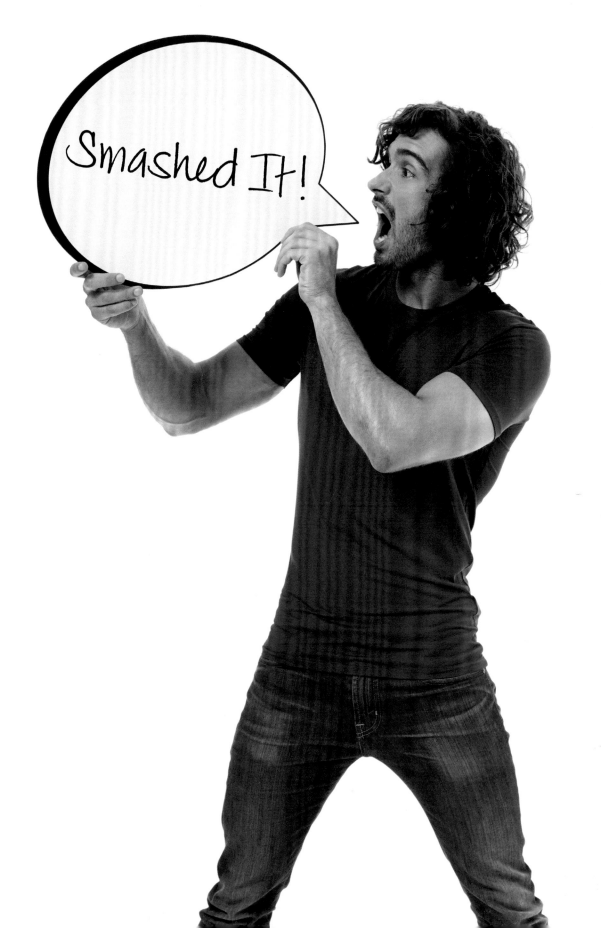

I've loved all the food and can't believe some of the portion sizes!

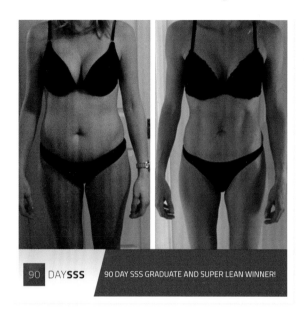

90 **DAYSSS** 90 DAY SSS GRADUATE AND SUPER LEAN WINNER!

★ 'Can't believe I've done it! I'm so pleased with my results. 16lbs down and 16 inches gone. I have stuck to the plan 100 per cent with both the food and exercise and haven't had any alcohol in over three months, but will now be having one to celebrate! I was a "fat thin" person and hated my tummy after having my children. My aim was just to be leaner: never in a million years did I think I'd be on my way to getting a six-pack and muscles! I soon got the hang of the plan. My first HIIT nearly killed me, but week by week I felt myself getting fitter and now, I love burpees! In cycles two and three I pushed myself with the weights and aimed to lift heavier each week, which I did, if only by 1kg. I've done all my workouts from home – I just bought some dumbbells and a barbell and used Joe's HIITs on YouTube, and a timer app on my phone. Much cheaper than a gym membership! At times I could have cried thinking I couldn't do it – this is as much a mental challenge as a physical one – but again, I pushed myself to achieve my goal. I've loved all the food and can't believe some of the portion sizes! Food prep is definitely key. I had a shocking diet before, which consisted of toast, biscuits, chocolate and a lot of takeaways. No wonder I always felt so ill! Until starting this plan, I'd never eaten anything green, other than a mint aero! But now I know what to eat and when and how important it is to fuel your body and not starve yourself.' Emma

" You have to be committed; you will only get out of it what you put in! "

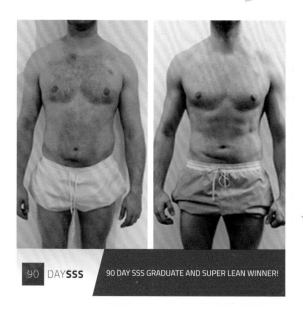

90 DAY**SSS**   90 DAY SSS GRADUATE AND SUPER LEAN WINNER!

★ 'So the end is here! I have been following Joe since the beginning and watched as his empire has grown. I always wanted to do it, but always found an excuse not to sign up (holidays, birthdays, Christmas, etc). I finally decided to take the plunge after becoming a father for the first time. It has been tough, both physically and mentally, with a few wobbles along the way, but 95 per cent of the time, I stuck to it. All the way through I kept thinking, "I can't wait to start eating normally again," but after three months, this is now normal! My girlfriend has been having similar meals to me and loves them as well, so we bought the *Lean in 15* cookbook and will be continuing with it now the plan has finished. It does change the way you look at food and at the diet industry as a whole. Mainstream media have been promoting the wrong ways to lose weight for years with under-eating and "detox" liquid diets (detox: isn't that what your kidneys do every day?), which are short-term plans designed to get you going back for more once the weight goes back on. This plan is different. I loved the workouts (despite avoiding cardio for years), especially once weights were introduced. I would highly recommend the plan to people, but you have to be committed to it; you will only get out of it what you put in!' Tommy

I feel so much stronger and healthier and happier

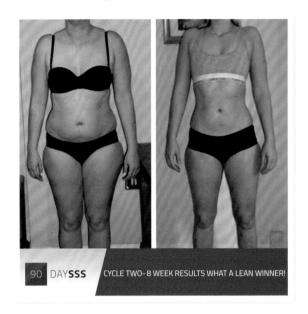

90 DAY**SSS**   CYCLE TWO- 8 WEEK RESULTS WHAT A LEAN WINNER!

★ 'Cycle two has been amazing. I was nervous about starting with the added carbs, however it's been fantastic! I have absolutely loved the weight training and learning what I can push myself to at the gym! I feel so much stronger and healthier and happier! I have stuck to it 100 per cent and it's been so much easier than I thought.' Daniella

If I can find the time to exercise and eat properly, anyone can

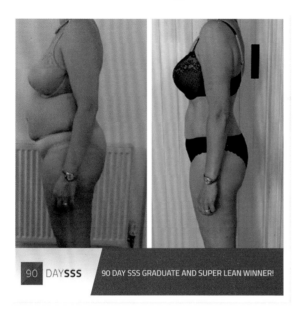

90 DAYSSS   90 DAY SSS GRADUATE AND SUPER LEAN WINNER!

★ 'Thank you, Joe Wicks, you have saved me from my midlife crisis! I was one hundred days from my fortieth birthday and my aim was not to be fat and forty . . . I have done it! I cannot believe my results. I have gone from a size 18 down to a 12, losing a total of 28.5 inches and 2 stone 4 lbs. I have totally changed the way I eat and think about food. I am crazy enough to say I am addicted to HIIT workouts. I have two small children and own a pub, and if I can find the time to exercise and eat properly, anyone can. So excited now to hit my forties!' Joanna

> **I now know what my body needs in order to be fuelled properly and I've gained confidence in my ability and appearance**

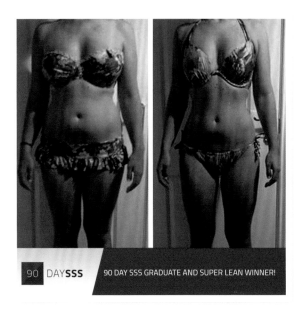

90 | DAY**SSS**   90 DAY SSS GRADUATE AND SUPER LEAN WINNER!

★ 'I followed Joe on social media for around a year before I decided to sign up. I had done a lot of his HIIT sessions on YouTube and found them more challenging than my usual gym routine. I was feeling bloated and was getting injured easily during my gym and running sessions. I decided to sign up to educate myself and tone up, rather than with the intention of losing weight. I couldn't believe that twenty minutes' exercise could burn off all the food I was eating. Previously I had eaten much less and exercised a lot more. The weights were brilliant. I could feel myself getting stronger every week, to the point where I matched my body-pump instructor on my squat weights (he was not happy!). Cycle three was probably my favourite because I was in a routine, I no longer felt like I was spending a lot of time prepping and I loved how much the exercise challenged me. It's not a diet and it's not a quick fix, but the results aren't just visual and that's the reason I signed up: I now know what my body needs in order to be fuelled properly and I've gained confidence in my ability and appearance.' Leanne

❝ I am finally seeing a difference in my body ❞

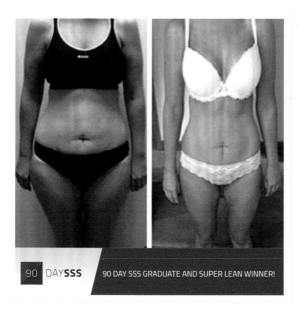

90 DAY**SSS** | 90 DAY SSS GRADUATE AND SUPER LEAN WINNER!

★ 'After having three children, one of whom was only nine months old when I started the plan, I am finally seeing a difference in my body and I am so glad I signed up to this. Thank goodness! Doing it with my husband meant we could give great support to each other. Bring on cycle three . . . I can't wait to see the end results.' Jillian

❛ This plan has truly been life-changing for me ❜

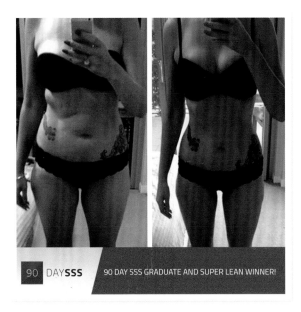

90 **DAYSSS**   90 DAY SSS GRADUATE AND SUPER LEAN WINNER!

★ 'I MADE IT!!!! I have spent years on diet after diet dreaming of the body I wanted but never reaching my goal. This plan has truly been life-changing for me. My progress cannot just be measured in inches and kgs, the true progress can be seen through my energy levels, my love of the gym and my passion for healthy food. This has taught me so many things. It's funny to think I'm eating more than I did but looking and feeling miles healthier and fitter. I have enjoyed every minute of this cycle and I can't wait to continue this as a lifestyle. But first, where's that champagne!' Emma

> ❝ As Joe says, this is a lifestyle change, not a diet ❞

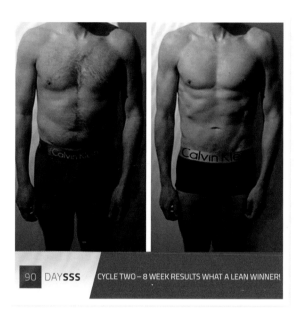

90 DAY**SSS** CYCLE TWO – 8 WEEK RESULTS WHAT A LEAN WINNER!

★ 'I have enjoyed the food on cycle two and I feel physically stronger and also enjoyed the training. This cycle is something I would like to continue after I graduate. I have certainly noticed a difference in myself, though I did have a couple of weekends where I relaxed; as Joe says, this is a lifestyle change, not a diet. The only regret I have is that I didn't sign up to the plan earlier as it's certainly given me more confidence. Let's see what cycle three brings.' Lewis

LEAN IN 15 HEROES

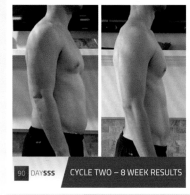

90 DAYSSS CYCLE TWO – 8 WEEK RESULTS

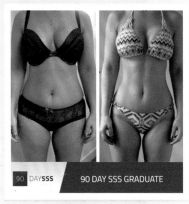

90 DAYSSS 90 DAY SSS GRADUATE

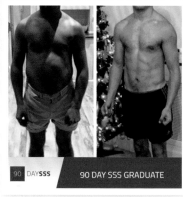

90 DAYSSS 90 DAY SSS GRADUATE

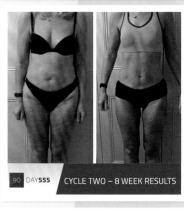

90 DAYSSS CYCLE TWO – 8 WEEK RESULTS

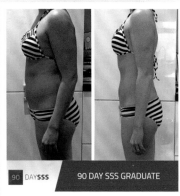

90 DAYSSS 90 DAY SSS GRADUATE

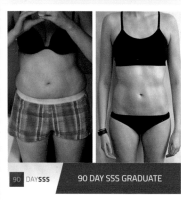

90 DAYSSS 90 DAY SSS GRADUATE

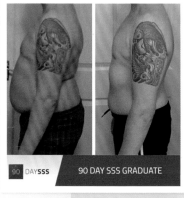

90 DAYSSS 90 DAY SSS GRADUATE

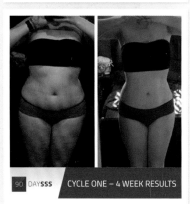

90 DAYSSS CYCLE ONE – 4 WEEK RESULTS

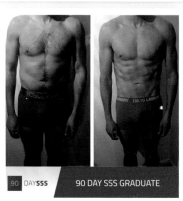

90 DAYSSS 90 DAY SSS GRADUATE

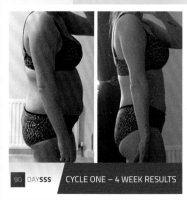

90 DAYSSS CYCLE ONE – 4 WEEK RESULTS

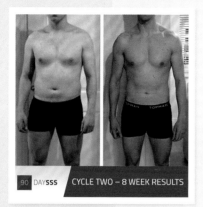
90 DAY**SSS** — CYCLE TWO – 8 WEEK RESULTS

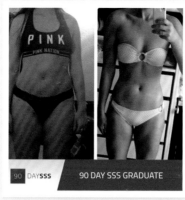
90 DAY**SSS** — 90 DAY SSS GRADUATE

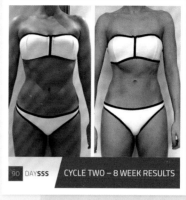
90 DAY**SSS** — CYCLE TWO – 8 WEEK RESULTS

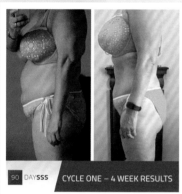
90 DAY**SSS** — CYCLE ONE – 4 WEEK RESULTS

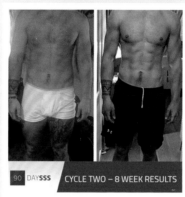
90 DAY**SSS** — CYCLE TWO – 8 WEEK RESULTS

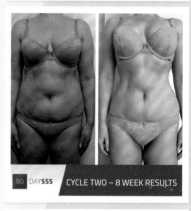
90 DAY**SSS** — CYCLE TWO – 8 WEEK RESULTS

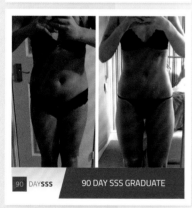
90 DAY**SSS** — 90 DAY SSS GRADUATE

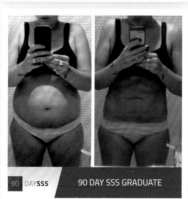
90 DAY**SSS** — 90 DAY SSS GRADUATE

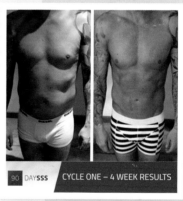
90 DAY**SSS** — CYCLE ONE – 4 WEEK RESULTS

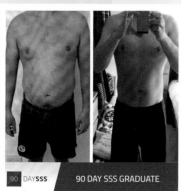
90 DAY**SSS** — 90 DAY SSS GRADUATE

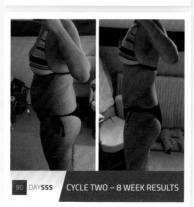
90 DAY**SSS** — CYCLE TWO – 8 WEEK RESULTS

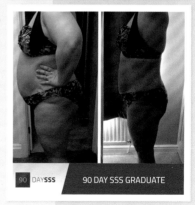
90 DAY**SSS** — 90 DAY SSS GRADUATE

INDEX

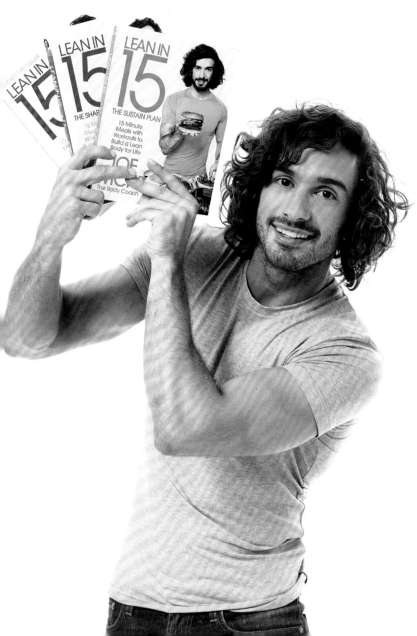

THE LEAN IN
15
TRILOGY
OUT NOW

ACKNOWLEDGEMENTS

I would like to say a huge thank you to everyone who has picked up one of my *Lean in 15* books or signed up to my 90 Day Shift, Shape and Sustain Plan. Thanks also for all your support on social media and for telling your friends about Lean in 15. It continues to help change people's lives for the better, so let's keep it going.

I also want to say a big thank you to my team at Bluebird, who have helped me produce three amazing books that I'm so proud of. Thanks Carole, Maja and Bianca for all your help in creating them.

Finally, I would like to dedicate this book to my brothers, Nikki and George, and my new nephew, Oscar Joseph Wicks. Everything I do in life is to make you proud and I know you've always got my back.

Love always,

Joe

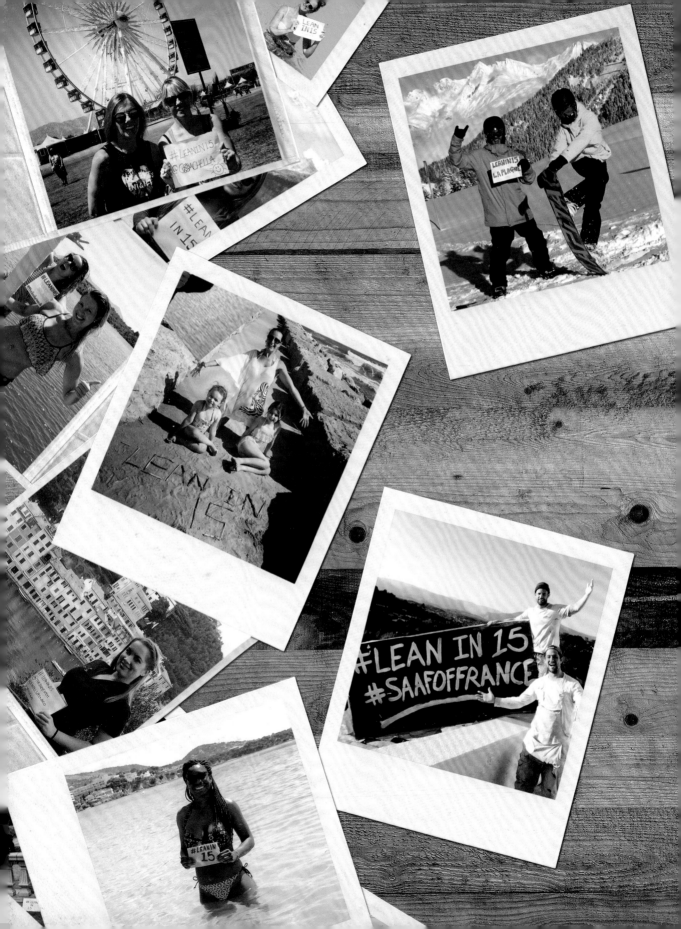

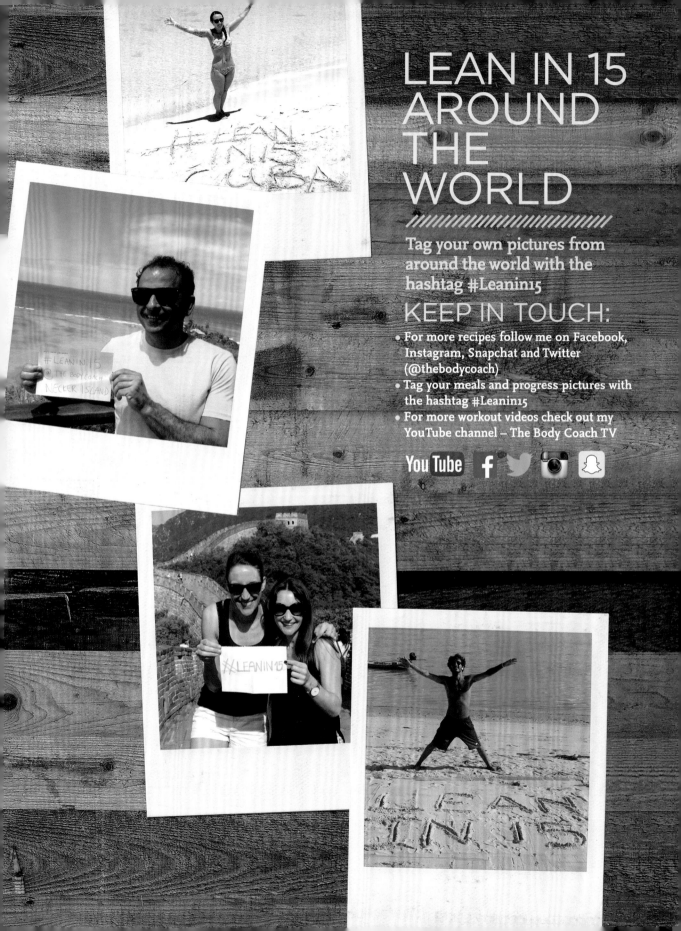

LEAN IN 15 AROUND THE WORLD

Tag your own pictures from around the world with the hashtag #Leanin15

KEEP IN TOUCH:

- For more recipes follow me on Facebook, Instagram, Snapchat and Twitter (@thebodycoach)
- Tag your meals and progress pictures with the hashtag #Leanin15
- For more workout videos check out my YouTube channel – The Body Coach TV

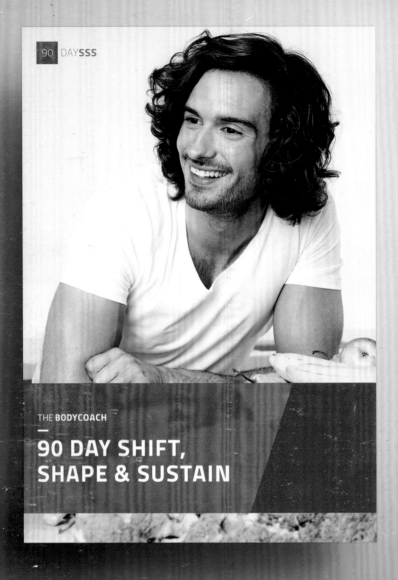

90 DAY**SSS**